BRITISH MEDICAL BULLETIN

VOLUME 53   NUMBER 2   199

Obesity

Scientific Editor

Nick Finer

Series Editors
P J Lachmann FRS FRCPath
L K Borysiewicz PhD FRCP

PUBLISHED FOR THE BRITISH COUNCIL BY
THE ROYAL SOCIETY OF MEDICINE PRESS LIMITED

ROYAL SOCIETY OF MEDICINE PRESS LIMITED
1 Wimpole Street, London W1M 8AE, UK
16 East 69th Street, New York, NY 10021, USA

British Library Cataloguing in Publication Data
A catalogue record for this book is available from the British Library
ISBN 1-85315-318-4
ISSN 0007-1420

Subscription information: *British Medical Bulletin* is published quarterly in January, April, July and October on behalf of the British Council by Royal Society of Medicine Press Limited. Subscription rates for Volume 53 (1997) are £134 Europe (including UK), US$222 USA, £137 elsewhere, £70 developing countries. Prices include postage by surface mail within Europe, by air freight and second class post within the USA*, and by various methods of air-speeded delivery to all other countries. Subscription orders and enquiries should be sent to: Publications Subscription Department, Royal Society of Medicine Press Limited, 1 Wimpole Street, London W1M 8AE, UK (Tel +44 (0)171 290 2928; Fax +44 (0)171 290 2929).
*Periodicals postage paid at Rahway, NJ. US Postmaster: Send address changes to *British Medical Bulletin*, c/o Mercury Airfreight International Ltd Inc, 2323 Randolph Avenue, Avenel, NJ 07001, USA.

Single copies (cased) and back numbers of issues published from 1996 are available at £45/US$73 and may be ordered from the Domus Medica, Royal Society of Medicine, 1 Wimpole Street, London W1M 8AE, UK (Tel +44 (0)171 290 2960; Fax +44 (0)171 290 2969); from booksellers; or directly from the distributors: Hoddle Doyle Meadows Limited, Station Road, Linton, Cambs CB1 6UX, UK (Tel +44 (0)1223 893855; Fax +44 (0)1223 893852).

Pre-1996 back numbers: Orders for any title published prior to 1996 should be sent to Pearson Professional Ltd, PO Box 77, Harlow, Essex CM19 5BQ, UK

This journal is indexed, abstracted and/or published online in the following media: Adonis, Biosis, BRS Colleague (full text), Chemical Abstracts, Colleague (Online), Current Awareness in Biological Science, Current Contents/Clinical Medicine, Current Contents/Life Sciences, Excerpta Medica/Embase, Index Medicus/Medline, Medical Documentation Service, Reference Update, Research Alert, Science Citation Index, Scisearch, SIIC-Database Argentina, UMI (Microfilms)

Phototypeset by Dobbie Typesetting Limited, Tavistock, Devon
Printed in Great Britain by Henry Ling Limited, The Dorset Press, Dorchester

BRITISH MEDICAL BULLETIN   Volume 53   Number 2   1997

Obesity

Scientific Editor

Nick Finer

Acknowledgements

The committee that planned this number of the *British Medical Bulletin* was chaired by Dr Nick Finer and included Ms Gill Cowburn, Dr Susan A Jebb, Dr Peter Kopelman and Professor Gareth Williams.

The British Council and Royal Society of Medicine Press are most grateful to them for their help and advice, and particularly to Dr Finer for his work as Scientific Editor.

Obesity — the inevitable penalty of civilisation?

Andrew M Prentice

MRC Dunn Clinical Nutrition Centre, Cambridge, UK

The modern inhabitants of 17th century cottages are reminded of the way in which the human form has changed every time they hit their head on a beam or stoop to pass through a doorway. The secular changes in the height of the Japanese over the past 50 years are an accelerated version of the same phenomenon. These are changes that we accept as being permanent and natural. We talk of 'reaching our genetic potential' in response to better nutrition, and view the changes as beneficial, since height is positively associated with health and social status. Are we now on the verge of another anthropometric transition — this time in weight? The evidence suggests that we are, but that this time the trend will be far from beneficial.

Data stretching back to the turn of the century show that the average body mass index (BMI = weight (kg)/height × height $(m)^2$) has increased steadily in the UK (where the best data are available) and other affluent countries. Such changes are graphically illustrated by the fact that Boeing's aeroplane designers have had to increase the assumed weight of each passenger by over 20 pounds since their first airliners took to the skies. Designers of clothes, and beds and chairs and cars, are all acknowledging that this increase in girth is not a temporary deviation in the statistics; it is here to stay and shows every sign of accelerating rapidly.

If left unchecked the future effects on society could be profound. In this book, Gill quotes Rose's statistical demonstration that when the mean weight of a population rises there comes a point when there is a sudden and disproportionate rise in the number of people who are seriously obese. The US passed this critical point some years ago and now has subgroups of the population (black, Hispanic and mid-American women) in whom the prevalence of clinical obesity exceeds 50%. Overseas visitors to the US will have no difficulty in reconciling these statistics with their own personal impressions, and will be struck by the massive, debilitating obesity that afflicts so many. The chapter by Seidell and Flegal shows that other affluent nations are close on the heels of the US, and that developing nations have no room for complacency especially among the urban rich.

In these days of political correctness, the gloomy tone of these predictions may appear hostile to the many self-help and self-protective organisations such as NAAFA (the North American Association for Fatness Acceptance) whose view is that the risks of obesity, and the

Correspondence to:
Dr Andrew M Prentice,
MRC Dunn Clinical
Nutrition Centre,
Hills Road, Cambridge
CB2 2DH, UK

benefits of weight loss are grossly overstated by a tyrannous medical profession bent on making their life a misery. This is a serious view, worthy of every sympathy, and it imposes on us a responsibility to critically examine the evidence of risk upon which we base our medico-centric attitudes.

Is obesity really harmful?

Jung's chapter provides an overview of the health risks of being obese, and the chapters by Kopelman & Albon and Pettigrew & Hamilton-Fairley examine two specific examples with illustrations of the likely mechanistic pathways.

Jung provides a condensed list of the morbidities associated with obesity. Even this shortened list runs to 45 diseases for which there is unequivocal statistical proof of increased risk. Among these are some of the biggest killers in modern societies including coronary heart disease, stroke, diabetes, and certain cancers.

Diabetes is one of the most thoroughly researched of the obesity-related syndromes and reveals some salutary messages. The incidence of new cases of NIDDM in previously healthy individuals has been carefully measured over an 8 year follow-up in over 50,000 middle-aged US male health professionals[1] and over a 14 year follow-up in over 110,000 US female nurses[2]. Body weight and weight change emerge as the most important predictors of the likelihood of developing diabetes with odds ratios rising to over 40-fold in men and over 90-fold in women who are seriously obese. Perhaps more worrying for health economists is the finding that the risk of NIDDM is significantly raised, by up to 8-fold, in people who are only mildly overweight.

Several arguments have been marshalled by those who wish to downplay the risks of obesity. The first is that some obese people are perfectly healthy; an argument which is extended to imply that it is something other than obesity which is causing illhealth. Of course some obese people are healthy, just as some 80-year-olds can run a marathon, a fact which does not disprove that ageing is associated with a general decline in physiological function. A corollary of this argument is the claim that obesity is not an *independent* risk factor for heart disease because it is displaced from regression analyses by other risk factors such as hypertension, hyperlipidaemia and hyperinsulinaemia. The fallacy inherent in this argument is the failure to accept that obesity is often the direct and pivotal cause of the hypertension, hyperlipidaemia and hyperinsulinaemia. A second argument has been that the curve for mortality is J-shaped with an increased risk among thin people as well as among fat people. As reported by Jung, this apparent excess risk among thin people has now been clearly shown to be due to an over-representation of smokers and people with pre-existing disease among the thin groups[3]. The third popular argument has been that the nadir of the mortality risk curve moves to the right (i.e. favouring fatter people) with increasing age, thus suggesting that it is natural and healthy to gain weight as we age. This claim has never been properly substantiated and is now largely discredited.

None of these arguments undermine the conclusion that serious obesity is seriously damaging to a person's health, and that mild obesity has a range of progressive effects on physiological function which ultimately cause a deterioration in health. Economic analyses as summarised by Hughes and McGuire suggest that the direct and indirect health costs attributable to obesity are around 5% of the total health budgets of affluent countries, equivalent to an astonishing $69 billion in the US.

These physical health effects are compounded by psychological and social burdens. Kolanowski's chapter on surgical interventions touches on the issue of quality of life for obese people, and records the benefits that many feel when they achieve substantial weight loss. The size of the benefit gives an indirect measure of the quality-of-life penalties borne by the seriously obese. Obese patients are reported to score worse than multiple amputees and tetraplegics on quality-of-life questionnaires. They have suffered a lifetime of bullying, social castigation and prejudice which result in prejudice and impaired opportunities in education, employment and marriage. Surveys in the US, during the 1970s, showed that obesity rated worse than a criminal conviction for rape as an undesirable feature in a potential marriage partner. Fortunately, these attitudes are now very different as a result of the effective lobbying by organisations such as NAAFA, and as a result of the fact that most people in the US now have at least one family member with obesity. The stigma is lessening, but the anguish remains acute for many sufferers.

Such a catalogue of side effects surely argues strongly in favour of a concerted, seriously-resourced national or international effort to combat the problem. But should we concentrate on prevention or cure? Can we effectively treat obese patients? And is it safe to do so? These issue are raised in the final chapters of this book. Let us first examine the question of safety.

Is weight loss beneficial?

Jung's chapter tabulates the benefits of a 10 kg weight loss, and shows substantial advantage in terms of co-morbidities and mortality. His interpretation is probably a balanced representation of current knowledge, but would not be universally accepted especially with respect to mortality. It has to be admitted that there are disquieting data available in the literature which still require explanation. For instance, the Harvard Alumni Study shows that weight stability is the optimal strategy for minimising coronary heart disease (CHD) and all-cause mortality, and that weight loss was associated with a *raised* mortality (even after allowing a considerable wash-out period to allow for deaths in people with pre-existing disease)[4]. Similar findings emerged from the NHANES follow-up studies[5], and there are repeated epidemiological surveys illustrating that weight-cycling (or yo-yo dieting) is associated with raised CHD mortality[6].

The defence that is usually mounted against these challenging findings is that they do not reflect the result of *intentional* weight loss achieved using modern dietary and pharmacological therapies. Some support for this claim is provided by recent analyses which do reveal reductions in mortality in people who intentionally and successfully lose weight[7].

In a similar vein of caution, we must also be careful not to assume that the obesity-related hypertension and insulin resistance carry the same mortality risks as hypertension and insulin resistance of other origin. It is known, for instance, that, although obesity is a major risk factor for hypertension, the incidence of stroke per case of hypertension is lower in the obese than in lean essential hypertensives[8]. We need new research to explore whether the physiological dysfunctions generated by obesity carry as much risk as the same dysfunction in a non-obese person. If this is not the case, it would support the view of those who believe that the risks have been exaggerated.

Can obesity be successfully treated?

Anyone working in this field will be familiar with Stunkard's famous adage that 'most obese people won't enter treatment, most who do won't lose weight, and most who lose weight regain it'. This nihilistic view is supported by statistics showing that the long-term cure rate for obesity is worse than for most forms of cancer.

Part of the explanation for such a poor treatment record lies with the fact that the statistics are derived from specialist tertiary referral centres which only receive the most severe cases; those who have failed all other attempts. In fact, broader community-based audits show that many people are very successful at long-term weight loss and management, but such people never appear in treatment statistics because they never seek formal treatment.

However, even allowing for this factor, the current treatment paradigms for obesity (with the possible exception of surgery) would not be described as successful by any truly impartial observer. The lifestyle and behavioural management strategies described by Cowburn, Hillsdon and Hankey are still in the infancy of their development as we start to learn some of the deeply-complex psychological factors underlying some obesities. The emerging pharmacotherapies described in Finer's chapter are likewise the first generations of drugs which will ultimately be much more effective. It is in this context that the new developments in neurobiology outlined in the chapter by Wilding, Widdowson and Williams may provide the vital insights into how we can ultimately design pharmacotherapies capable of disrupting the feeding drive which we are now learning has multiple fail-safe back-up systems.

But, even when such drugs are developed, we will be faced with some testing ethical and economic decisions. What will be the potential for abuse of such drugs by a population which is increasingly obsessed by their body image, and in which eating disorders are a major concern? Will we be able to afford to maintain a substantial proportion of the population on lifelong therapy? Is this the best way to allocate resources or should we focus on prevention?

Prevention or treatment — where should we prioritise?

Notwithstanding the compassionate need to help people who are already obese, there would be few analysts who would argue with the view that prevention of obesity is the only viable long-term strategy if we are seriously to tackle the problem. In this context, we need to understand the causes of the current epidemic before we can institute effective remedial measures. The chapter by Jebb analyses the likely aetiological factors.

On the one hand the search for causes seems impossible since energy balance only needs to be displaced by a tiny fraction for the cumulative effects to result in obesity. The fattest man in the world died recently in his mid-forties weighing 465 kg (73 stone). Even this enormous accumulation of fat required an excess equivalent to only a small bar of chocolate each day. The smaller changes characteristic of most obesities are, therefore, beyond the limits of detection of most metabolic measurements. This problem is reinforced by the now well known fact that it is virtually impossible to obtain an accurate record of habitual food intake in obese people because of the layers of psychoses and subconscious self-deception which have built up as a protection against social stigma.

However, the quest is not hopeless and certain useful observations can be made with some certainty. The first is that there are many different types of obesity ranging from the purely genetic (e.g. Prader–Willi syndrome) through the purely environmental (e.g. pastry cooks and sweet-shop owners) to the purely behavioural (e.g. Sumo wrestlers). Within this spectrum there are certain categories, such as sufferers of binge eating disorder, which are becoming clinically recognised as discrete aetiologies. There is an urgent need to progress our under-standing of the different phenotypes of obesity so that each can be targeted with appropriate therapeutic measures. The current approach, which often applies the same therapeutic methods to all patients, must be inefficient and may actually be harmful since some components, such as restrictive dieting, might actually reinforce some of the causal factors such as bingeing.

The second useful observation that can be made with certainty is that most modern obesities must be caused by environmental and lifestyle factors in modern life, since the epidemic is emerging within a relatively constant gene pool. This does not mean that genetic effects are unimportant; there is ample evidence to prove that some individuals, and some tribal groups, are more genetically susceptible than others, and the concept of the 'thrifty genotype' probably remains valid 30 years after it was initially proposed. But the balance of genetic versus environmental influences is changing. Figure 1 gives a schematic representation of what is happening. In the past, average BMI was around $21-22 \, kg/m^2$ and there was only a shallow right hand tail to the distribution pattern. Under such conditions it was highly likely that any seriously obese person would have a definite genetic susceptibility perhaps resulting from a single major gene defect, or more likely arising from a cluster of minor genetic variants. The situation has already moved to one in which the genuine genetic susceptibilities are being obscured by the sheer volume of lifestyle obesities. As more and more people become obese the concept of genetic susceptibility loses value, and attention will be turned to those who seem to be genetically resistant to weight gain.

Jebb's chapter identifies high-fat diets and physical inactivity as the prime aetiological candidates. High-fat diets have a high energy density and result in so called 'passive overconsumption' where people accidentally overconsume energy without necessarily eating a large bulk of food. Physiological studies show that human metabolism is very poorly adapted to recognise excess fat consumption and to re-establish fat balance. This effect interacts with physical inactivity such that the combination of inactivity and high-fat foods is especially adipogenic.

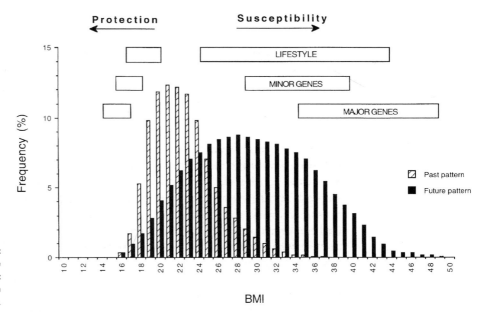

Fig. 1 A schematic illustration of the changing role of genetic and lifestyle influences on obesity.

Analysis of secular and cross-sectional epidemiological data from a variety of sources suggests that the physical inactivity characteristic of modern sedentary lifestyles is possibly the dominant factor in inducing obesity. This is key to the preventative strategies outlined by Gill and to the behavioural therapeutics outlined by Cowburn, Hillsdon and Hankey. The data in this area suggest that inactivity is not just the reciprocal of activity. It is often a specific trait, such as obsessive TV viewing, and one which is actively promoted by marketing of TV and video programmes, home computers, video games, and energy-sparing domestic devices. The increasing use of motorised transport, lifts and escalators, mobile telephones, central heating and so on, all conspire to save energy. Unfortunately, our physiological homeostatic mechanisms fail to detect this and to adequately down-regulate food intake with the result that the excess has to be stored as fat unless we use cognitive controls (restrained eating and/or exercising to maintain healthy weight) to take over from the fallible innate mechanisms.

Is there hope for the future?

It is easy to become demoralised by the enormity of the task involved in trying to reverse the current trends in obesity, but there is hope. At the extremes of obesity the present spate of 'gene-a-month' discoveries will soon have identified most of the major and minor genes involved in pathological weight gain. This will aid our understanding of the principles involved, help to develop improved pharmacotherapy, and perhaps even lead to gene therapies in the longer term. Advances in our understanding of the psychological aspects of obesity are also leading to greatly improved behavioural change models for treatment. The importance of an increased research effort into the fundamental causes of obesity cannot be overstated.

But at a more general societal level the omens are less encouraging. Whatever advice we offer in terms of environmental modifications always appears to be swimming against the rip tide of 'progress' which is backed by the enormous resources of global TV giants, motorcar manufacturers, multinational fast-food chains, and such like. Surely we will never stop this particular juggernaut. So the glimmer of hope lies in the fact that many individuals do in fact manage to maintain a lifetime's healthy weight in spite of living within such an obesogenic environment. Knowledge and motivation seem to be key elements of success, and the best riposte to those who claim that behavioural changes are ineffective comes from the observation that obesity shows a strong inverse correlation with level of education in most affluent countries.

We have elsewhere argued that increasing peoples' activity levels and reducing their fat intake are likely to be the critical components in successful weight management[9]. This advice is absolutely in line with recommendations emanating from other disease areas such as CHD, diabetes and cancer. There is a powerful synergism developing, and we now need to persuade the general public of the immense benefits to health and well-being that would accrue if they would adopt more healthy lifestyles. Education appears to be the only really viable option in tackling the current epidemic of obesity, but that education needs to be based on a solid foundation of knowledge about the causes and consequences of obesity of the type contained in the following chapters.

References

1 Chan J, Stampfer M, Rimm E, Willet W, Colditz G. Obesity, fat distribution, and weight gain as risk factors for clinical diabetes in men. *Diabetes Care* 1994; **17**: 961–9
2 Colditz G, Willet W, Rotnitzky A, Manson J. Weight gain as a risk factor for clinical diabetes mellitus in women. *Ann Intern Med* 1995; **122**: 481–6
3 Manson J, Willet W, Stampfer M *et al*. Body weight and mortality among women. *N Engl J Med* 1995; **333**: 677–85
4 Lee IM, Paffenbarger RS. Change in body weight and longevity. *JAMA* 1992; **268**: 2045–9
5 Pamuk E, Williamson D, Madans J *et al*. Weight loss and mortality in a national cohort of adults, 1971–1987. *Am J Epidemiol* 1992; **136**: 686–97
6 Muls E, Kempen K, Vansant G, Saris W. Is weight cycling detrimental to health? A review of the literature in humans. *Int J Obesity* 1995; **19** (**Suppl 3**): S46–S50

7   Williamson D, Pamuk E, Thun M *et al*. Prospective study of intentional weight loss and mortality in never smoking overweight US white women aged 40–64 years. *Am J Epidemiol* 1995; **141**: 1128–41

8   Barret-Connor E, Khaw K-T. Is hypertension more benign when associated with obesity? *Circulation* 1985; **72**: 53–60

9   Prentice AM, Jebb SA. Obesity in Britain: gluttony or sloth? *BMJ* 1995; **311**: 437–9

Assessing obesity: classification and epidemiology

Jacob C Seidell* and Katherine M Flegal[†]

*Department of Chronic Disease and Environmental Epidemiology, National Institute of Public Health and the Environment, Bilthoven, The Netherlands; [†]National Center for Health Statistics, Centers for Disease Control and Prevention, Hyattsville, Maryland, USA

Obesity is generally defined as a body mass index (BMI) of 30 kg/m² and higher. Overweight is defined as a BMI between 25 and 30 kg/m². The prevalence varies considerably between countries, and between regions within countries. It is estimated that more than half of adults aged 35–65 living in Europe are either overweight or obese. Overweight is more common among men than among women but obesity is more common among women. The prevalence of obesity in Europe is probably in the order of 10–20% in men and 15–25% in adult women. In most European countries who have reliable data on time-trends the prevalence of obesity seems to be increasing. In most European countries, obesity is usually inversely associated with socio-economic status, particularly among women. New classifications of overweight may be based on cut-off points for simple anthropometric measures which reflects both total adiposity as well as abdominal fatness.

How to measure obesity

Correspondence to:
Dr Jacob C Seidell,
Department of Chronic
Disease and
Environmental
Epidemiology, National
Institute of Public Health
and the Environment,
PO Box 1,
3720 BA Bilthoven,
The Netherlands

When we speak about the prevalence of obesity in populations we actually mean the fraction of people who have an excess storage of body fat. In adult men with an average weight, the percentage body fat is in the order of 15–20%. In women this percentage is higher (about 25–30%). Because differences in weight between individuals are only partly due to variations in body fat, many people object to the use of weight or indices based on height and weight (such as the body mass index, BMI) to discriminate between overweight and normal weight people. There are always examples which illustrate the inappropriate use of body mass index in certain individuals, such as an identical body mass index in a young male body builder and a middle aged obese women. However, despite these obvious extremes, there is a very good correlation between BMI (weight divided by height squared) and the percentage of body fat

Table 1   Cut–off points proposed by a WHO Expert Committee for the classification of overweight[3]

Body mass index	WHO classification	Popular description
$< 18.5 \, \text{kg/m}^2$	Underweight	Thin
$18.5–24.9 \, \text{kg/m}^2$	—	'Healthy', 'normal' or 'acceptable' weight
$25.0–29.9 \, \text{kg/m}^2$	Grade 1 overweight	Overweight
$30.0–39.9 \, \text{kg/m}^2$	Grade 2 overweight	Obesity
$\geqslant 40.0 \, \text{kg/m}^2$	Grade 3 overweight	Morbid obesity

in large populations. Deurenberg *et al.*[1] established that one can quite accurately estimate the body fat percentage in adults with the following equation:

Body fat%=1.2 (Body Mass Index)+0.23 (age) − 10.8 (gender) − 5.4

where gender=1 for men and gender=0 for women.

About 80% of the variation in body fat between (Dutch) individuals could be explained by this formula. The standard error of estimate was about 4%. It follows from this equation that, for a given height and weight, the body fat percentage is about 10% higher in women compared to men. In addition, people get fatter when they get older even when their body weights are stable. The good correlation between BMI and fat percentage implies that, in populations, BMI can be used to classify people in terms of excess body fat. In practice, people or populations are usually not classified on the basis of the body fat percentage but on the basis of their BMI. Usually, the same cut-off points are applied for men and women and for different age groups. This is done because the relationships between BMI and mortality are similar (i.e. the relative mortality associated with obesity is similar in men and women, in most age groups the absolute mortality is much lower). The same relative risk and lower absolute risk associated with overweight and obesity among women compared to men implies that women can probably tolerate body fat better than men. The reason in women could be that their excess body fat is usually distributed as subcutaneous fat and mainly peripherally (thighs, buttocks, breasts) and in men there is a relative excess of body fat stored in the abdominal cavity and as abdominal subcutaneous fat. It has been suggested that optimal BMI (i.e. the BMI associated with lowest relative risk) increases with age[2]. The reasons why older people seem to tolerate an excess body fat better than younger people are manifold, and range from selective survival to decreased lipolysis of adipose tissue in older people. The cut-off points have recently been proposed by a WHO Expert Committee for the classification of overweight (Table 1)[3]. These figures apply to both men and women and to all adult age-groups. There are limitations in the interpretation of body mass index in very old subjects as well as in certain ethnic groups with deviating body proportions (e.g. in populations where stunted growth is common, in those with relatively short leg length compared to sitting height).

How to measure fat distribution

Since the pioneering work of Jean Vague in the 1940s, it has slowly become accepted that different body morphology or types of fat distribution are independently related to the health risks associated with obesity[4]. Starting with Jean Vague's brachio-femoral adipo-muscular ratio as an index of fat distribution (which was based on ratios of skinfolds and circumferences of the arms and thighs), more recent indices have been adopted to predict specifically intra-abdominal fat. The most popular among all measures is the waist/hip circumference ratio. The simplest of these measures is the waist circumference, which has been suggested to predict intra-abdominal fat at least as accurately as the waist/hip ratio[5] and to predict levels of cardiovascular risk factors and disease as well as BMI and waist/hip ratio[6]. It has also been suggested that waist circumference could possibly be used to replace classifications based on BMI and the waist/hip circumference ratio[7]. More complex measures, such as the sagittal abdominal diameter, the ratio of waist/thigh circumference, the ratio of waist/height or the conicity index, have also been proposed to perform even better than waist circumference for one or more of these purposes. However, the differences among these measures are small and the use of ratios may complicate the interpretation of associations with disease and their consequences for public health measures. For instance, the waist/height ratio may be a better predictor of morbidity because the waist is positively associated with disease and because height, for reasons unrelated to body composition or fat distribution, is inversely associated with disease.

Replacing BMI and waist/hip ratio by simple cut-off points which are optimal for each sex, age group, population and relationship with specific diseases may, however, be too simple. Still, as suggested by Lean

Table 2 Sex-specific cut-off points for waist circumference. Level 1 was initially based on replacing the classification of overweight (BMI $\geqslant 25\,kg/m^2$) in combination with high waist/hip ratio (WHR $\geqslant 0.95$ in men and $\geqslant 0.80$ in women). Level 2 was based on classification of obesity (BMI $\geqslant 30\,kg/m^2$) in combination with high waist/hip ratio[6,7]

	Level 1 ('alerting zone')	Level 2 ('action level')
Men	$\geqslant 94\,cm$ (~ 37 inches)	$\geqslant 102\,cm$ (~ 40 inches)
Women	$\geqslant 80\,cm$ (~ 32 inches)	$\geqslant 88\,cm$ (~ 35 inches)

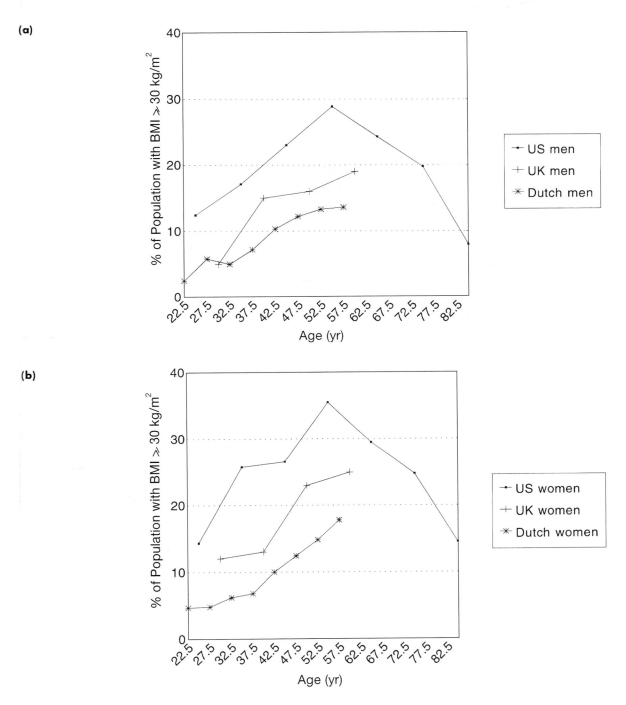

Fig. 1 (a) and (b)   Prevalence of obesity (BMI > 30 kg/m²) in men (A) and women (B) by age in the US (NHANES III, 1988–1994), in the UK (national survey 1992) and in The Netherlands (about 13000 people measured in 1993–1995 in three towns).

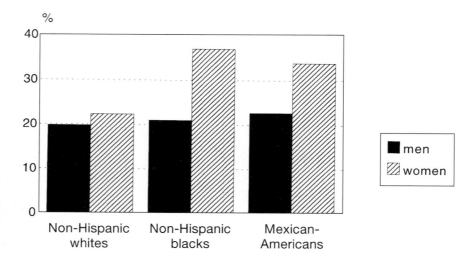

Fig. 2 Prevalence of overweight (BMI > 30 kg/m²) in different race–ethnic groups in the US in 1991 (midpoint of NHANES III).

et al.[7], some cut-off points may be of guidance in interpreting values of waist circumference for adults (Table 2). Other cut-off points, based on classification of subjects on a 'critical level' of intra-abdominal fat, have been proposed by investigators from Quebec[8].

Who is obese?

Very little is known about the factors that may explain the large differences between populations in the distributions of BMI (see next section). Obviously, overweight in individuals in any population is the result of a long-term positive energy balance. Just to say that overweight is characterised by physical inactivity or ingestion of large quantities of food is an oversimplification. Several epidemiological studies have shown that the following factors are associated with overweight in the population.

Demographic factors

Age: overweight increases with age, at least up till age 50–60 years in men and women. Figure 1a,b shows the relation between age and prevalence of obesity in the UK (1992 data), The Netherlands (1993–1995 data) and the USA (NHANES III 1988–1994)[9–11].

Gender: women have generally higher prevalences of obesity compared to men especially when older than 50 years of age.

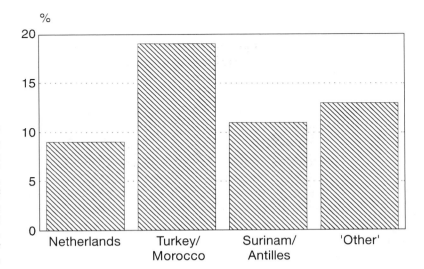

Fig. 3 Prevalence of obesity in 4450 children aged 4–15 years living in The Netherlands in 1993/1994 according to the 97th percentile values of BMI for age in French children (Rolland Cachera *et al.*, 1982). Stratified by nationality of the father.

Ethnicity: there are large, usually unexplained, variations between ethnic groups. Figure 2 shows that in the US there is little variation for men by race–ethnic group but much larger differences for women by race–ethnic group. Figure 3 shows the prevalence of overweight among Dutch children by ethnic group and illustrates the higher prevalence among children of immigrants compared to 'native' Dutch children[12].

Socio-cultural factors

Educational level and income: in industrialized countries, there is a higher prevalence of overweight in those with lower education and/or income.

Marital status: Usually overweight increases after marriage.

Biological factors

Parity: it has been claimed that BMI increases with increasing number of children, but recent evidence suggests that this contribution is, on average, likely to be less than 1 kg per pregnancy. Many study designs confound the changes in weight with aging and parity.

Behavioural factors

Dietary intake: although it is clear that nutrition is of critical importance in establishing a positive energy balance, research on this topic has not been easy to interpret because of confounding factors including increased under-reporting with increasing degrees of obesity. Another reason may be that only small deviations in energy balance are necessary to yield large differences in body weight in the long term. The methodological errors in determining energy intake may be too large to allow detection of the nutritional determinants of obesity. In particular, the fat percentage of the diet has been proposed to be associated with higher prevalence of obesity, although also on this topic the epidemiological evidence may be flawed or biased[13].

Smoking: smoking lowers body weight and cessation of smoking increases body weight. The associations between smoking and obesity may, however, vary considerably among populations[14].

Alcohol consumption: the effect is unclear in most populations. Moderate alcohol consumption is sometimes associated with higher body mass index.

Physical activity: those who remain or become inactive are usually heavier then those who are physically active. Similar limitations apply as for the interpretation of the evidence of nutritional determinants of obesity: methodological problems, such as confounding and biased reporting as well as measurement error, make it difficult to interpret the literature.

Prevalence of obesity in Europe

Obesity, defined as a body mass index greater than 30 kg/m², is a common condition in Europe and the US[15]. In order to make a comparison possible between countries, it is necessary to compare population-based data on measured height and weight in which identical protocols for measurement were applied and which were collected in the same period. The most comprehensive data on the prevalence of obesity in Europe are from the WHO MONICA study[16]. Most of these data were collected between 1983 and 1986. The populations studied, however, do not necessarily represent the population as a whole.

Tables 3 and 4 show the age-standardised prevalence of overweight and obesity in 39 European centres participating in this study[16]. Only in

Table 3 Prevalence of overweight (BMI 25–30 kg/m^2) and obesity (BMI $\geqslant$ 30 kg/m^2) in European men aged 35–64 years. Data from the WHO MONICA (first round 1983–1986) populations[16]

Country	Center	Prevalence		
		Overweight	Obese	Overweight+obese
Iceland	Iceland	44	11	55
Sweden	Northern Sweden	45	12	57
Sweden	Gothenburg	44	7	51
Finland	Kuopio Province	50	18	68
Finland	North Karelia	51	17	68
Finland	Turku-Loima	49	19	68
Denmark	Glostrup	44	11	55
UK	Glasgow	46	11	57
UK	Belfast	45	11	56
Germany	Bremen	53	14	67
Germany	Rhein-Neckar	52	14	66
Germany	Augsburg	56	18	74
Germany	Augsburg (rural)	56	20	76
Germany	Halle County	51	18	69
Germany	Karl-Marx-Stadt	50	15	65
Germany	Cottbus County	51	17	68
Germany	'Rest of DDR MONICA'	54	19	73
Belgium	Ghent	50	11	61
Belgium	Charleroi	48	20	68
Belgium	Luxembourg Province	45	14	59
France	Lille	44	14	58
France	Bas Rhin/Strassbourg	52	22	74
France	Haute Garonne/Toulouse	51	9	60
Switzerland	Vaud-Fribourg	49	12	61
Switzerland	Ticino	51	19	70
Russia	Novosibirsk (2 samples)	46	14	60
Russia	Moscow (2 samples)	45	13	58
Lithuania	Kaunas	54	22	76
Poland	Warsaw	48	17	65
Poland	Tarnobrzeg Voivodship	39	13	52
Czech Rep.	'Czechoslovakia'	51	21	72
Hungary	Pecs	42	19	61
Hungary	Budapest	46	15	61
Serbia	Novi Sad	50	18	68
Spain	Catalonia	57	9	66
Italy	Area Brianza	44	11	55
Italy	Friuli	49	17	66
Italy	Area Latina	52	18	70
Malta	Malta	46	25	71
95% CI of mean		46.2–51.4	14.2–16.8	62.1–66.3
Mean $\pm$ SD		48.8 $\pm$ 4.1	15.5 $\pm$ 4.2	64.2 $\pm$ 6.8

three centres was the prevalence of obesity slightly lower than 10% (Gothenburg, Sweden (men and women); Toulouse, France (men); Catalonia, Spain (men)) and, on average, the prevalence of obesity was about 15% in men and 22% in women. Overweight, on the other hand, is much more common among men than among women. More than half

Table 4 Prevalence of overweight (BMI 25–30 kg/m²) and obesity (BMI ⩾ 30 kg/m²) in European women aged 35–64 years. Data from the WHO MONICA (first round 1983–1986) populations[16]

Country	Center	Prevalence		
		Overweight	Obese	Overweight+obese
Iceland	Iceland	30	11	41
Sweden	Northern Sweden	33	14	47
Sweden	Gothenburg	25	9	34
Finland	Kuopio Province	39	20	59
Finland	North Karelia	37	23	60
Finland	Turku–Loima	37	17	54
Denmark	Glostrup	25	10	35
UK	Glasgow	38	16	54
UK	Belfast	34	14	48
Germany	Bremen	37	18	55
Germany	Rhein–Neckar	31	12	43
Germany	Augsburg (urban)	36	15	51
Germany	Augsburg (rural)	36	22	58
Germany*	Halle County	36	25	61
Germany*	Karl-Marx-Stadt	31	19	50
Germany*	Cottbus County	36	23	59
Germany*	'Rest of DDR MONICA'	35	27	62
Belgium	Ghent	37	15	52
Belgium	Charleroi	35	26	61
Belgium	Luxembourg Province	33	18	51
France	Lille	30	18	48
France	Bas Rhin/Strassbourg	34	23	57
France	Haute Garonne/Toulouse	25	11	36
Switzerland	Vaud–Fribourg	30	12	42
Switzerland	Ticino	29	14	43
Russia	Novosibirsk (2 samples)	38	44	82
Russia	Moscow (2 samples)	39	34	73
Lithuania	Kaunas	38	45	83
Poland	Warsaw	39	26	65
Poland	Tarnobrzeg Voivodship	36	32	68
Czech Rep.	'Czechoslovakia'	37	31	68
Hungary	Pecs	34	26	60
Hungary	Budapest	36	18	54
Serbia	Novi Sad	40	30	70
Spain	Catalonia	44	24	68
Italy	Area Brianza	28	15	43
Italy	Friuli	37	19	56
Italy	Area Latina	43	30	73
Malta	Malta	32	41	73
95% CI of mean		33.2–36.0	18.8–24.6	52.5–60.1
Mean ± SD		34.6 ± 4.5	21.7 ± 9.1	56.3 ± 12.2

of the people aged 35–65 years in Europe seem to be either overweight or obese. Given the large within and between-country estimates of the prevalence of obesity, it is difficult to derive an overall prevalence figure for Europe as a whole from these data. It is fairly safe to assume that such an overall prevalence figure would be in the range of 10–20% in men and 15–25% in women.

The study of explanations for the large diversity in prevalence data could give important clues to the understanding of the origins of common obesity. For example, the very high prevalence of obesity and mean body mass indexes in women from Eastern European countries is striking. There is only a moderate association ($r=0.39$, $P=0.02$) of the prevalence of obesity between men and women[17]. The distributions of the BMI values in men seem to be rather homogeneous over Europe, despite large socio-economic and cultural differences between the countries. In addition, it is clear that there are major differences in the mortality rates of cardiovascular disease which, at least in men, cannot be explained by differences in body mass index[17].

Table 5 Recent trends in obesity prevalence in some European countries and the US

Country	Obesity definition (BMI cut-off point)	Year	Ages	Men %	Women %
England	30 kg/m^2	1980	16–64	6	8
		1986/7		7	12
		1991		13	15
		1993		13	16
Sweden	Men: 30 kg/m^2	1980/1	16–84	4.9	8.7
	Women: 28.6 kg/m^2	1988/9		5.3	9.1
Finland	30 kg/m^2	1978/9	20–75	10	10
		1985/7		12	10
		1991/3		14	11
Germany	30 kg/m^2	1985	25–69	15.1	16.5
		1988		14.7	17.2
		1990		17.2	19.3
East Germany	30 kg/m^2	1985	25–65	13.7	22.2
		1989		13.4	20.6
		1992		20.5	26.8
The Netherlands	30 kg/m^2	1987	20–59	6.0	8.5
		1988		6.3	7.6
		1989		6.2	7.4
		1990		7.4	9.0
		1991		7.5	8.8
		1992		7.5	9.3
		1993		7.1	9.1
		1994		8.8	9.4
		1995		8.4	8.3
US	30 kg/m^2	1960/2	20–74	10.0	15.0
		1971/4		11.6	16.1
		1976/80		12.0	14.8
		1988/94		19.7	24.7

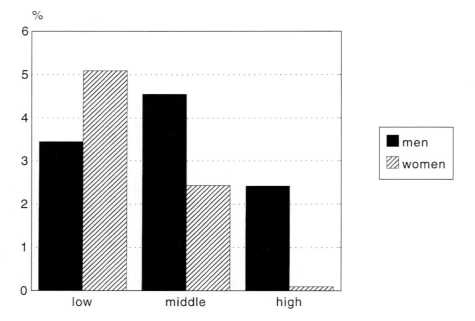

Fig. 4 Changes in prevalence of obesity (in percent over the period 1987–1995) in three Dutch towns by educational level (previously unpublished data). Low=primary education and lower vocational training; middle = secondary education and higher vocational training; high=tertiary education.

Trends in obesity prevalence in Europe and the US

Table 5 shows some of the available recent trend data on obesity in Europe and the US. The prevalence has increased by about 10–40% in most countries in the past decade. It escalated in the UK, where the prevalence has doubled during this period.

It seems that, in most countries, obesity is increasing in prevalence, although preliminary data from Denmark[18] show that in the period 1960–1980, the prevalence increased in men and decreased in women.

Subgroup analyses by sex, age and educational level with regard to time-trends yield different results in different countries. In some studies, the increase in the prevalence of obesity is most pronounced in young adults, whereas in others it is more pronounced in older subjects. Usually, there is a greater increase in the prevalence of obesity in those with relatively low educational levels compared to those with higher education. Figure 4 illustrates, with data from The Netherlands, that changes in body mass index may differ according to level of education.

National surveys in the US have shown a marked increase in the prevalence of obesity over time. During 1960–1980, there was only a slight increase in overweight. However, between 1980 and 1994 a striking increase in the prevalence of overweight occurred. This increase was seen for all age groups, for both men and women, and for non-Hispanic whites, non-Hispanic blacks and Mexican-Americans. The magnitude of the increase was similar for all these groups. The US experience shows that a population-wide increase in the prevalence of overweight may occur relatively quickly after a long period during which the prevalence of overweight is fairly stable.

Causes of time trends in obesity

Diminished physical activity, high fat diets and inadequate adjustments of energy intakes to the diminished energy requirements are likely to be major determinants of the observed changes. Prentice and Jebb[19] have proposed that, on a population level, limited physical activity may be more important than energy or fat consumption in explaining the time-trends of obesity in the UK. Their analysis was based on surrogate measures of physical activity (such as number of hours spent watching television) and household consumption survey data. Such data are open to bias. Energy and fat consumption are selectively under-reported with increasing degrees of overweight[13]. Changes in smoking behaviour may also contribute to changes in body weight on a population level. Data from the US show that, although smoking cessation could explain some of the increase in the prevalence of overweight, smoking cessation alone could not account for the major portion of the increase[20]. In other studies it was also shown that the increase in obesity prevalence may be independent of smoking status[21,22].

Epidemiological methods that can be used to assess energy intake and energy expenditure not only may be subject to bias, but also have a high ratio of within to between-subject variation. It should be noted that only small changes in energy balance are needed to increase average BMI by one unit and, depending on the distribution of BMI in the population, could greatly increase the prevalence of obesity. Such small changes in energy balance may not be detectable by epidemiological measures of energy expenditure and intake.

It was previously shown[23] that dramatic increases in the prevalence of obesity in The Netherlands (about 37% in men and 18% in women over a period of 10 years) can be the consequence of relatively minor changes in average body weight. If height had remained constant, an average weight increase of only slightly less than 1 kg over 10 years could account for the increased prevalence of obesity observed. Such a small increase could reflect a minute change in energy balance on a daily basis. Experimentally, overfeeding with about 7,000 kcal will result in a weight gain of, on average, about 1 kg. If we neglect all metabolic adaptations to overfeeding and increases in body weight, we can calculate that a constant positive energy balance of about 2 kcal/day may be sufficient to increase the average body weight of individuals by about 1 kg in 10 years and thus result in a substantial increase in the prevalence of obesity. It is clear that such small persistent changes in energy balance are not detectable by existing methods for measuring energy expenditure and energy intake in populations.

In The Netherlands, data from two identical nutrition surveys performed in 1987–1988 and 1993 suggested that energy intake decreased from 2329 kcal/day (9746 kJ) in 1987–1988 to 2216 kcal/day (9278 kJ) in 1993[24]. This reduction of about 113 kcal/day was attributable to a decrease in fat consumption (protein intake increased and carbohydrate and alcohol consumption remained constant). Smoking behaviour had changed, particularly in men, since the 1970s, but in the 1980s no further decrease was observed. This may imply that daily energy expenditure has decreased during the same period with the same order of magnitude. It is not uncommon in societies which are in a phase of 'post-modernisation' to see simultaneous improvement in dietary intakes (reduction in fat and energy) and increases in the prevalence of obesity[13].

Conclusions

Overweight and obesity are common in Europe and the US and, in most countries where reliable data are available, the prevalence seems to be increasing. Targets to reduce the prevalence of obesity to acceptable levels will not be reached in most countries[25,26]. International guidelines for the treatment and, in particular, the prevention of obesity are urgently needed[27]. They should be aimed at groups at high risk for weight gain. These include those who have a genetic predisposition for weight gain and obesity, but also those who change their life style (e.g. those who stop smoking or those who reduce their physical activity) and, perhaps, women who become pregnant. Special targets should be developed to reach specific socio-economic and ethnic groups which have a high prevalence of obesity. Efforts to prevent excessive weight gain in children and adolescents should be balanced against the possibility of inducing unnecessary dieting behaviour and eating disorders in girls.

Promoting physical activity is a priority in this context and attention should not just be focused on more participation in sports clubs but should also stimulate normal outdoor activities, such as walking and cycling and discouragement of 'sedentary behaviour'. International guidelines, such as those prepared by the International Task Force on Obesity[27], can only be implemented when sufficient input and commitment of governments and health professionals have been obtained.

References

1 Deurenberg P, Weststrate JA, Seidell JC. Body mass index as a measure of body fatness: age- and sex-specific prediction formulas. *Br J Nutr* 1991; **65**: 105–14

2 Andres R. Mortality and obesity: the rationale for age-group specific weight-height tables. In: Andres R, Bierman EL, Hazzard WR (eds) *Principles of Geriatric Medicine*. New York: McGraw Hill; 1985: 311–8

3 WHO Expert Committee. *Physical Status: the use and interpretation of anthropometry*. WHO Technical Report Series no. 854. Geneva: WHO, 1995

4 Vague J. The degree of masculine differentiation of obesity — a factor determining predisposition to diabetes, atherosclerosis, gout and uric calculus. *Am J Clin Nutr* 1956; **4**: 20–34

5 Pouliot MC, Despres JP, Lemieux SL *et al*. Waist circumference and abdominal sagittal diameter: best simple anthropometric indexes of abdominal visceral adipose tissue accumulation and related cardiovascular risk in men and women. *Am J Cardiol* 1994; **73**: 460–8

6 Han TS, van Leer EM, Seidell JC, Lean MEJ, Han TS. Waist circumference action levels in the identification of cardiovascular risk factors: prevalence study in a random sample. *BMJ* 1995; **311**: 1401–5

7 Lean MEJ, Han TS, Morrison CE. Waist circumference indicates the need for weight measurement. *BMJ* 1995; **311**: 158–61

8 Lemieux S, Prud'homme D, Bouchard C, Tremblay A, Despres J-P. A single threshold value of waist girth identifies normal-weight and overweight subjects with excess visceral adipose tissue. *Am J Clin Nutr* 1996; **64**: 685–93

9 Department of Health. *The Health of the Nation: one year on... a report on the progress of the Health of the Nation*. London: HMSO, 1993

10 Seidell JC. Lichaamsgewicht. In: Maas I *et al*. (eds) *Determinanten van Gezondheid*. VTV, 1997; In press

11 Flegal KM, Carrol MD, Kuczmarski RJ, Johnson CL. Prevalence and trends in grades 1, 2, and 3 overweight in the United States. Submitted for publication

12 Brugman E, Meulmeester JF, Spee-van der Wekkes J, Beuker RJ, Radder JJ. *Peilingen in de jeugdgezondheidszorg: PGO-peiling 1993/1994*. TNO Preventie en Gezondheid, report nr. 95.061

13 Seidell JC. Dietary fat and obesity: an epidemiological perspective. *Am J Clin Nutr* 1997; In press

14 Molarius A, Seidell JC, Kuulasmaa K, Dobson A, Sans S. Smoking and body weight: WHO MONICA Project. *J Epidemiol Community Health* 1997; In press

15 Seidell JC. Obesity in Europe —scaling an epidemic. *Int J Obesity* 1995; **Suppl. 3**: S1–S4

16 WHO MONICA Project. Risk factors. *Int J Epidemiol* 1989; **18 (Suppl. 1)**: S46–S55

17 Seidell JC, Rissanen N. Global prevalence of obesity and time trends. In: Bray GA, Bouchard C, James WPT (eds) *Handbook of Obesity*. New York: Dekker, 1997; In press

18 Mikkelsen KL, Heitmann BL, Sörensen TIA. Secular changes in mean body mass index and its prevalence of obesity — three Danish population studies of 31,000 subjects (Abstract). *Int J Obesity* 1995; **19 (Suppl. 2)**: 30

19 Prentice AM, Jebb SA. Obesity in Britain: gluttony or sloth? *BMJ* 1995; **311**: 437–9

20 Flegal KM, Troiano RP, Pamuk ER, Kuczmarski RJ, Campbell SM. The influence of smoking cessation on the prevalence of overweight in the United States. *N Engl J Med* 1995; **333**: 1165–70

21 Boyle CA, Dobson AJ, Egger G, Magnus P. Can the increasing weight of Australians be explained by the decreasing prevalence of cigarette smoking? *Int J Obesity* 1994; **18**: 55–60
22 Wolk A, Rössner S. Effects of smoking and physical activity on body weight: developments in Sweden between 1980 and 1989. *J Intern Med* 1995; **237**: 287–91
23 Seidell JC. Time trends in obesity: an epidemiological perspective. *Horm Metab Res* 1997; In press
24 Voorlichtingsbureau voor de Voeding. *Zo eet Nederland 1992: Resultaten van de Voedselconsumptiepeiling 1992*. Den Haag, 1993
25 Smith SJL. Britain is failing to meet targets on reducing obesity. *BMJ* 1996; **312**: 1440
26 Russel CM, Williamson DF, Byers T. Can the year 2000 objective for reducing overweight in the United States be reached? A simulation study of the required changes in body weight. *Int J Obesity* 1995; **19**: 149–53
27 Woodman R. WHO launches initiative against obesity. *Lancet* 1996; **347**: 751

A review of the economic analysis of obesity

David Hughes and **A McGuire**

Department of Economics, City University, London, UK

There are indications that the treatment costs arising from obesity are significant. However, the cost-of-illness studies undertaken to date also highlight two other important points. First, the cost of treatment is sensitive to the body mass index (BMI) cut-off used. Given that there is no definitive definition of obesity as based on BMI, a range of costs reflecting differing BMI cut-offs may be more appropriate than the use of a single figure. Second, the costs are, not surprisingly, also sensitive to the defined associated diseases. Again there is little agreement on these and also little information on the relative risks of attributable diseases arising from obesity. The calculations of the cost-of-illness arising from the treatment of obesity, and its associated conditions must, therefore, remain indicative rather than authoritative.

Correspondence to:
Dr David Hughes,
Department of
Economics,
School of Social Sciences,
City University,
Northampton Square,
London EC1V 0HB, UK

Obesity is a common health problem which is a recognised disease in its own right, but also a major risk factor for a number of other diseases, including cardiovascular disease, non-insulin dependent diabetes, certain cancers, gallbladder disease and hypertension. Normally measured through the use of the body mass index (BMI), obesity has been classified as a BMI above $30 \, kg/m^2$. The risk of associated disease increases with BMI. There is also evidence that obesity decreases longevity[1,2].

The number of obese individuals in the UK has also been increasing over the past 10–15 years. Recent data have estimated the percentage of individuals who are obese as 13% for men and 16% for women in the UK, although for overweight and obesity, individuals with a BMI above $25 \, kg/m^2$, the percentages increase to 57% and 48%, respectively[3,4]. The impact of the disease is, therefore, liable to increase in the future with a consequent rise in the resources drawn to its treatment. Given the prevalence of the disease, it is perhaps surprising that little analysis of the resource consequences have been undertaken. The aim of this paper is to undertake a review of the economic studies applied to obesity. As we shall discover, there is a very thin literature on this subject matter and most of this is not, strictly speaking, concerned with economic evaluation. Prior to discussing the specific literature it is, then, worthwhile defining some of the different types of economic analysis.

Types of economic analysis

It is increasingly obvious that resources devoted to health care are scarce and limited. While the encouragement of a more rational use of health resources should be welcomed by all, there are concerns that quality might be sacrificed in order to control cost. Yet it is precisely because economic analysis is based on an assessment of both costs and benefits that it is a tool that allows the relative merits of alternative resource usage to be appropriately considered. Thus, economic efficiency is not the same as cost cutting. In many cases, the key issue of economic evaluation is whether additional benefits justify the additional costs. Indeed, when the overall level of resources is limited, cost and benefit are the opposite sides of the same coin. If the health care budget is fixed, more costs in some parts of the health-care system mean that benefits are forgone elsewhere. Efficiency is then determined by the relative costs and benefits derived from different allocations.

Economic evaluation of health care is the generic term referring to the various methods used to make the costs and benefits associated with any change in health service delivery explicit. These methods consider the costs of health care interventions and their consequences. If a new health care technology is introduced, both the relative benefits and the relative costs of that technology are calibrated against existing treatment. If the benefits to be gained from the new intervention were no greater than those already achieved by the existing treatment, yet the costs were higher, economic evaluation would reject the introduction of the product on the grounds of inefficiency. Conversely, if the benefits were at least as good as those achieved by existing health technology and the costs were lower, economic evaluation would advocate the introduction of the new intervention on efficiency grounds. Where the benefits and the costs of the new technology are both higher or both lower, the argument for introduction on efficiency grounds depends on the degree and rate at which health benefits.

Economic evaluation provides a means to adjudicate between the relative costs and benefits arising from competing health care technologies. However, a form of analysis which, while not an economic analysis but nevertheless does involve quantification of resource use, is the 'burden of illness' or 'cost of illness' method.

Burden of illness or cost of illness studies are not particularly common in the disease area of obesity. They are a separate form of analysis, not to be confused with economic evaluation, which quantifies the existing burden imposed on society, or cost to society, of a given disease. They do not consider the relative costs and consequences derived from new treatment technologies. **Burden of illness** and **cost of illness** studies estimate the absolute amount of resources used in treating a disease over a given period. They are not concerned with evaluating the resource impact of a new form of treatment, but give an indication of the full cost (measured in terms of mortality and morbidity as well as treatment resource costs) imposed by a disease on society. These studies indicate the current total cost of treating a particular disease as part of their analysis. They may be prevalence or incidence based.

There are a number of specific forms of **economic evaluation** which differ in the extent to which they measure and value the consequences. Otherwise the analysis is much the same: each formulation attempts to consider the cost of achieving particular consequences. All economic evaluations consider costs. All are based on the comparison of different treatment programmes. Different techniques address different questions. The question to be addressed determines the technique to be employed. The different approaches are defined as follows.

Cost-minimisation analysis

All forms of economic evaluation consider the costs arising from the use of resources to achieve therapeutic outcomes. Only one form of analysis, **cost-minimisation analysis**, considers costs alone. It is relevant, there-fore, only when the medical effects of two alternative therapies are identical, such as in the substitution of an equivalent generic product for a branded one. If the interventions do not have identical outputs in terms of health gain, then cost-minimisation is not a form of economic evaluation. Rather it is reduced to a simple analysis of the costs of alternative treatments. Unfortunately, all too often, outcomes are ignored and costs alone are minimised, as in a number of so-called 'efficiency saving' exercises which are, in effect, budgetary control measures. This may be good accounting practice, it is not good economic practice.

Cost-effectiveness analysis

Few interventions reduce costs overall and usually the assessment of an intervention compares the resource input with the improvements in health obtained. Another form of analysis, **cost-effectiveness analysis**, assesses the consequences of treatment intervention in the most convenient natural units, normally some physical measure of the health care output associated with treatment. Common measures of effects relate to physiological measures taken from clinical trial data, for example changes in BMI could be used. It is important, however, to consider the validity of the units of effect used, as they may not correlate well with health gain.

Alternative common measures of effectiveness are the number of 'symptom-free' or 'disease-free' days, if morbidity is influenced by treatment. If mortality is affected by treatment, changes in survival probabilities (normally converted through the use of life tables to changes in life expectancy or, even more commonly, life-years gained) may be used as a measure of effectiveness.

Cost-utility analysis

In many situations, it is important to consider also the preferences of individuals towards different forms of intervention. The preferences of individuals reflect the gain in welfare or satisfaction or, to use a more unfashionable term, the utility arising from the treatment. **Cost-utility analysis** attempts to do so by attaching preference values to the outputs associated with treatment. While cost-utility analysis does not fully value the health gains associated with interventions, in that it stops short of attaching monetary valuation to outcomes, it does move in the direction of a fuller definition of the benefits derived from health care by incorporating information on preferences.

The preference information is used as a weighting of the physical output measure which forms the basis of the cost-effectiveness analysis. The most common form of cost-utility analysis to date has been based on the measure of outcome from health care in terms of the quality of the life-years gained. Here, preference valuations on different levels of quality of life are used to weight changes in survival probabilities associated with interventions. Results are then presented in terms of cost per quality adjusted life-year (QALY) gained from alternative treatments.

Quality of life is also important for those chronic conditions where therapy adds life to years rather than years to life. Evaluation assessing the benefits in quality-adjusted life-years are called cost-utility analyses. As cost-utility analysis does not consider the full value of the intervention it is again concerned with productive efficiency. Although, as the health gain is measured in commensurate units, QALYs, there is scope for comparisons across different forms of intervention.

Cost-benefit analysis

There have been few comprehensive cost-benefit analyses where attempts are made to assess all the costs and benefits in monetary terms. The advantage of **cost-benefit analysis** is that there is direct measurement of the valuation individuals themselves attach to the health benefit, and both costs and benefits are measured by a commensurate instrument – money. This allows direct comparison across all forms of intervention and provides information on the most highly valued uses of health care resources. Thus, direct information is made available to allow the optimal mix of health outputs to be provided. Not surprisingly, however, it is particularly difficult to assess health benefits in monetary terms. The general approach is to estimate the value in monetary terms of the full impact of an intervention. This is normally addressed through trying to elicit the willingness to pay for a change in health state arising from a particular treatment or intervention.

Each form of evaluation adopts a similar approach. Cost-benefit analysis compares the opportunity costs associated with achieving treatment outcomes with a quantitative measure of the value of the benefits achieved. Cost-effectiveness analysis and cost-utility analysis each attempts to quantify the total resource cost and the total outcome (weighted outcome in the case of cost-utility analysis) associated with a pre-specified intervention and compare these with the total cost and the total outcome achieved from the next best use of resources. Cost-benefit analysis requires no comparator intervention, while both cost-effective-ness and cost-utility analysis do.

In order to facilitate such comparison, cost-effectiveness and cost-utility analysis are normally presented as a ratio with the total cost divided by the total outcome achieved to give a cost per unit of outcome. The lowest cost per unit of outcome is the most productively efficient intervention. Subsequently, the cost per life year gained is calculated by dividing the total costs arising from an intervention by the total calculated life years gained from an intervention. In comparing two, or more, interventions, the one achieving the lowest cost per life year saved is the most productively efficient allowing a given budget to buy the greatest level of output.

Economic studies of obesity

As noted above, there have been very few economic studies in this disease area. Possibly the most comprehensive coverage to date has been the reportage of a seminar in a special edition of *PharmacoEconomics* (Vol. 5, Suppl., 1994) and the reporting of a set of conference papers in a supplement to the *International Journal of Obesity* (Vol. 19, Suppl. 6, 1995). Like most other studies, these papers mainly were concerned with the cost of illness rather than comparisons of the economic efficiency of different interventions to control obesity. Most of the studies concentrated on the direct costs imposed on the health system arising from the current prevalence and treatment of the disease. The simplest manner in which this could be undertaken is to estimate the treatment prevalence of obesity for specified treatments in a specific health care system and then attach unit costs of the individual treatments to gain an estimate of the aggregate cost of obesity. This would, however, certainly underestimate the costs borne by health care systems, as it is well established that obesity leads to an increased risk of co-morbidity in other diseases. To estimate the cost of direct treatment of obesity, the cost of treating these co-morbidities as attributable to obesity must be estimated. This has been approached in a number of manners.

The simplest approach is that adopted by Colditz[5] in a US study. Colditz first identified the relevant co-morbidities as cardiovascular disease (CVD), gallbladder disease and cholcystectomy, colonic and postmenopausal breast cancer, hypertension and non-insulin dependent diabetes. The cost of treatment of each of these co-morbidities attributable to obesity was calculated by assuming that a given amount of the disease is diagnosed amongst obese individuals of which a certain proportion is attributable to obesity. He then used estimates of the aggregate costs of treating the identified co-morbidities by applying this proportion to an estimate of the cost of treating co-morbid diseases in the attributable population. For example, Colditz[5] assumes 27% of CVD is diagnosed in obese individuals and that, among the obese, 70% of CVD is attributable to obesity. Thus 19% (0.27×0.70) of the estimated aggregate cost of treating CVD in the US can be attributed to the disease obesity. Overall, the costs attributed to obesity were $22.2 billion arising from CVD, $2.4 billion for gallbladder disease, $1.9 billion for colonic and breast cancer, $1.5 billion for hypertension and $11.3 billion for non-insulin dependent diabetes. This gives an estimate of $39.3 billion as the cost of treating obesity in the US in 1986. Extending the definition of co-morbidities somewhat, for example by including musculoskeletal diseases, and up-dating these earlier calculations, Wolf and Colditz[6] revised the estimate of the direct cost of treating obesity in the US to be $45.8 billion in 1990. To put this in perspective, this amounted to approximately 6% of the total expenditure on health care in the US in 1990.

Using a similar approach, West[7] estimated the treatment cost arising from obesity in the UK to be around £195 million, of which the cost of treating obesity directly was around 15% (£29.35 million). He estimated that a further £85.5 million was spent through the purchase of dietary products.

More rigorous calculations of the attributable costs arising from treating co-morbidities are given in Levy et al.[8], Segal et al.[9], and

Seidell[10]. These calculations are similar to the calculations used by epidemiologists to estimate attributable risk, which is defined as the proportionate excess risk of disease that is associated with exposure to a risk factor. Using obesity as the risk factor, population attributable fractions (PAFs) were first calculated by Segal et al[9]. These are the product of the relative risk (rr) and the prevalence risk factor (P):

$$PAF = P(rr-1)/[P(rr-1) + 1)]$$

This is precisely the same expression as that calculated by Levin[11] for attributable risk. Given information on the relative risk of disease in obese patients, the PAF can be calculated to estimate direct cost of treating obesity; this is based on the excess population in the co-morbid conditions attributed to have the condition as a result of obesity and then the proportion of costs of treating these co-morbidities that ought to be attributed to these conditions. Segal et al.[9] used the same information on co-morbidities as reported in Colditz[5] and estimated the total cost of treating obesity in Australia in 1989 as $A395 million. Of this, approximately 7% ($A28.7 million) are costs which are incurred as a result of treating obesity itself, with the vast majority of costs resulting from the treatment of co-morbidity. As in the Colditz studies, hypertension and CVD were the most significant co-morbidities in terms of cost.

Levy et al.[8] used a much more extensive range of co-morbidities but applied the same methodology based on attributable risk. They estimated that the direct cost of treating obesity in France in 1990 was approximately FFr12 billion or approximately 2% of the French health care costs. This was based on information relating to relative risks arising from a BMI $>27 \, kg/m^2$. Their study showed that, if the calculations were based on a BMI $>30 \, kg/m^2$, the costs fell to FFr5.8 billion, highlighting that the estimated cost of treatment is sensitive to the BMI cut-off used.

Seidell[10] used a similar methodology to report the direct costs of treating overweight and obese patients for their condition and associated conditions in The Netherlands. Overweight is defined as being present if individuals have a BMI $>25 \, kg/m^2$ but $<30 \, kg/m^2$, and obesity is defined as a BMI $>30 \, kg/m^2$. It was estimated that the cost of treatment of both overweight and obese individuals amounted to around 4% of the total Dutch health care costs; obesity itself accounts for about 1% of the total costs of health care. From this, and the studies by Levy et al.[8] and Segal et al.[9], Seidell estimated that, depending on the definition of obesity, the cost impact of treating this condition and its attributable co-morbidities is between 1% and 5% of total health care costs[10].

Using a different methodology based on a regression model, Hakkinen[12] estimated the excess use of health care in Finland due to obesity. A latent variable model was constructed to assess the impact of obesity on health and, through this, on health care utilisation. The model estimated that if all Finns could be reduced to normal body weight, i.e. a BMI $<25 \text{ kg/m}^2$, then 190 million Finnish marks could be saved from the health care budget; cessation of smoking by all Finns was estimated to save 150 million Finnish marks in the same model.

Concentrating on a specific medical event, Galtier-Dereure et al.[13] found that, during pregnancy, obesity caused many more complications than in a control group. Moreover, the mean duration of hospitalisation and cost were significantly correlated with maternal weight. The results were based on a retrospective study of 112 deliveries from 89 overweight and obese women during 1980–1993 and compared with a control group of 54 normal weight women over the same period. They found, for example, that 66% of massively obese (BMI $<35 \text{ kg/m}^2$), 36% of obese (BMI $30\text{–}35 \text{ kg/m}^2$) and 33% of overweight (BMI $25\text{–}30 \text{ kg/m}^2$) pregnant women were hospitalised compared with 9% in the control group. Overall cost was 3 times higher in the massively obese than in the normal weight women. Moreover, about two-thirds of infants born to obese mothers required care in a paediatric unit.

As well as the direct costs arising from the treatment of obesity, a number of studies have calculated the indirect costs of the disease. The direct costs may be defined as any costs arising as a direct result of treatment intervention. These are commonly restricted to health care costs but could include, for example, costs incurred by patients themselves; hence slimming or dietary amendment costs incurred by the individual are direct costs. Indirect costs are the costs which impose further effects, arising from the presence of a disease, on sectors other than the health care sector. The most obvious example is the cost resulting from obesity when individuals have to take time off work as a result of the disease. This results in a loss of productive output and is a cost to society. This is, of course, a restricted notion of indirect cost. There may be considerable social and psychological costs arising from obesity which are recognised but never quantified (for a fuller discussion see Gorstein and Grosse[14] and Hutton[15]).

Colditz[5] estimated the indirect costs arising from lost productivity to be $20 billion for the US in 1986 and $23 billion in an up-dated paper[6]. Sjostrom et al.[16], using survey material, estimated that the level of sickness absence was 1.4–2.4 times higher in obese patients than in normal weight individuals and the number on disability pension was 1.5–2.8 times higher. Extrapolating to the Swedish population as a whole, they estimated that 7% of total productivity loss in Sweden was obesity related. Generally, however, indirect costs are estimated to be considerably lower than the direct costs of treating obesity and associated diseases.

This limited evidence would imply that the cost of treating obesity is a major draw on resources. Whether this resource impact can be alleviated by better or more comprehensive treatment is unknown as there has been little proper economic evaluation of the treatment of obesity. Beales and Kopelmen[17] give an overview of the existing available methods of treating obesity, but note that there is little evidence on the success of the various interventions in controlling weight loss. Detailed costing information on the various interventions is also not readily available. Thus, it is not surprising that there are extremely few true economic evaluations of the treatment of obesity.

Dahms *et al.*[18] conducted a study of the cost-effectiveness of behavioural therapy (consisting of group discussions led by a dietician), placebo and two anorectic drug regimens in a population of 120 obese patients over a 14 week period. One of the problems in establishing effectiveness in obesity arises from compliance: indeed, in this particular study, only 33 patients completed the programme. All treatment groups lost similar amounts of weight, and there was no significant difference between the placebo and either of the drugs (mazindol and diethylpropion). Given this and adverse effects recorded with the drug regimens, behaviour therapy was recommended to be the most cost-effective practice.

Martin *et al.*[19] compared the cost-effectiveness of medical and surgical treatment of severely obese individuals. The mean BMI for surgical patients was $49.3\,kg/m^2$ and for medical patients it was $41.2\,kg/m^2$. The study included 464 subjects who were monitored for 2–6 years over the period 1984–1991: 362 patients completed the programme. A total of 201 patients were entered into the surgical programme, Roux-en-Y gastric bypass, and 161 entered into the medical programme, weekly meetings for 1.5 years with dietary and life-style advice. Successful completion was taken to mean a loss of one-third of excess weight above ideal body weight. The economic end point was the cost per pound lost. The cost per pound lost was recorded at each follow-up point. Over the whole period, the medical programme had a marginally more cost-effective impact; however, by the sixth post-treatment year, the cost per pound lost for the medical treatment exceeded that of the surgical treatment. On this basis, the authors concluded that the surgical intervention was more cost-effective, but this may not be the correct conclusion. For example, it is unclear precisely what time period is being considered. Six years of follow-up were reported, but no explanation as to why this period had been decided on. Moreover, it is not clear that the costs had been discounted. If they had been, then over the follow-up period reported it is probable that the medical management would have been more cost-effective than the surgical intervention.

Discussion

Given that these costs do appear to be significant in most health care systems, it is perhaps surprising that there have been so few economic evaluations of the existing treatments. For any economic evaluation, however, there has to be reliable clinical evidence of efficacy at least. Accepting the difficulties associated with measuring long term follow-up, not least the high withdrawal rates to be expected in this area, the lack of economic evaluation could reflect the low level of clinical evidence in this disease area. As reported, we have only been able to trace two such evaluations, both of which are cost-effectiveness studies. Given the impact that obesity has on an individual's perception of well being, it is perhaps also surprising that there have been no economic evaluations based on quality of life measures. We can only hope that, as we drift away from the *Health of the Nation* targets in this area, more effort will be concentrated on the effective strategies to control obesity and that the cost-effectiveness of these strategies will be considered.

References

1 Lew E, Garfinkel L. Variations in mortality by weight among 750,000 men and women. *J Clin Epidemiol* 1979; **32**: 563–76

2 Manson J, Stampfer MJ, Hennekens CH *et al*. Body weight and longevity: a reassessment. *JAMA* 1987; **257**: 353–9

3 Breeze *et al*. *The Health of the Nation*. Department of Health (OPCS Social Survey Division), Series HS 2. London: HMSO, 1994

4 *Health Survey for England 1993*, Series HS no. 3. London: HMSO, 1995

5 Colditz G. Economic costs of obesity. *Am J Clin Nutr* 1992; **55**: 503S–507S

6 Wolf A, Colditz G. The cost of obesity: the US perspective. *PharmacoEconomics* 1994; **5** (**Suppl. 1**): 34–7

7 West R. *Obesity*. Office of Health Economics Monographs on Current Health Issues, no 112. London: Office of Health Economics, 1994

8 Levy E, Levy P, LePen C *et al*. The economic cost of obesity: the French situation. *Int J Obes* 1995; **19**: 788–92

9 Segal L, Carter R, Zimmet P. The cost of obesity: an Australian perspective. *PharmacoEconomics* 1994; **5** (**Suppl. 1**): 45–52

10 Seidell J. The impact of obesity on health status: some implications for health care costs. *Int J Obes* 1995; **19** (**Suppl. 6**): S13–S16

11 Levin ML. Attributable risk. *Acta Unio Int contra Cancrum* 1953; **9**: 531–5

12 Hakkinen U. The production of health and the demand for health care in Finland. *Soc Studies Sci* 1991; **33**: 225–37

13 Galtier-Dereure F, Montpeyraux F, Boulot P *et al*. Weight excess before pregnancy: complications and costs. *Int J Obes* 1995; **19**, 443–8

14 Gorstein J, Grosse R. The indirect cost of obesity. *PharmacoEconomics* 1994; **5** (**Suppl. 1**): 58–61

15 Hutton J. The economics of treating obesity. *PharmacoEconomics* 1994; **5** (**Suppl. 1**): 66–72

16 Sjöström, Larsson B, Backman L *et al*. Recruitment for an intervention study and a selected description of the obese state. *Int J Obes* 1992; **16**: 465–79

17 Beales P, Kopelmen P. Management options in obesity, *PharmacoEconomics* 1994; **5** (**Suppl. 1**): 18–32

18 Dahms W, Molitch M, Bray A *et al*. Treatment of obesity: a cost-benefit analysis of behavioral therapy, placebo and two anorectic drugs. *Am J Clin Nutr* 1978; **31**: 774–8

19 Martin L, Tan T, Horn J *et al*. Comparison of the costs associated with medical and surgical treatment of obesity. *Surgery* 1995; **118**: 599–607

Aetiology of obesity

Susan A Jebb

MRC Dunn Clinical Nutrition Centre, Cambridge, UK

Obesity is not a single disorder but a heterogeneous group of conditions with multiple causes each of which are ultimately expressed as an obese phenotype. Fatness does run in families, but the genetic component does not follow simple Mendelian principles and the influence of the genotype on the aetiology of obesity may be attenuated or exacerbated by non-genetic factors. Body weight is ultimately determined by the interaction of genetic, environmental and psycho-social factors acting through the physiological mediators of energy intake and expenditure.

Aetiological determinants of obesity

Endocrine and hypothalamic disorders

A number of endocrinological disorders may contribute to obesity, although these represent only a very small proportion of the total cases. The endocrinological determinants of obesity have recently been reviewed[1]. The most common single disorder in this group is hypothyroidism in which weight gain occurs primarily as a consequence of decreased energy expenditure. Others include Cushing's syndrome and disorders of corticosteroid metabolism, where weight gain is accompanied by characteristic patterns of fat deposition in the truncal region, sex hormone disorders including hypogonadism in men and ovariectomy in women, insulinoma and growth hormone deficiency. Here weight gain is believed to occur predominantly due to increases in energy intake. The polycystic ovarian syndrome of Stein–Leventhal is commonly associated with obesity which may be related to altered ovarian function or hypersensitivity of the hypothalamic-pituitary-adrenal axis.

Hypothalamic tumours or damage to this part of the brain as a consequence of irradiation, infection or trauma may also lead to obesity, apparently due to a defect in appetite control and subsequent hyperphagia. However, altered hypothalamic control of the autonomic nervous system may also reduce energy requirements in these patients. A

Correspondence to:
Dr Susan A Jebb,
MRC Dunn Clinical
Nutrition Centre,
Hills Road, Cambridge
CB2 2DH, UK

hypothalamic disorder is also believed to be the origin of a number of congenital abnormalities which result in obesity, e.g. Prader–Willi syndrome.

Genetic considerations

Heritability   At a population level, the genetic component of obesity is expressed in terms of heritability. This refers to the proportion of the total variation in a character which is attributable to genetic factors. The heritability of obesity may be considered either in terms of the total fatness of an individual or the distribution of body fat.

Numerous studies in different ethnic groups suggest that the familial correlation in total body fatness, expressed as body mass index, (BMI; kg/m^2) from parent to offspring is about 0.2 and for sibling–sibling relationships about 0.25[2,3]. As would be expected, studies of twins show a much higher correlation, particularly for monozygotic pairs. However, these findings do not segregate the independent effects of genetic transmission and a shared environment. Further studies of twins reared apart attribute 50–70% of the difference in BMI in later life to genetic factors[4,5]. Adoption studies, where an individual is compared both to their biological and adopted parents, have also demonstrated the importance of genetic influences. There is a strong relationship between the BMI of the adoptee and their biological parents across the entire range of fatness, but no relationship between the adoptee and their adoptive parents[6,7].

Studies of fat distribution have considered both the ratio of subcutaneous to total fat mass and the distribution of subcutaneous fat in the trunk relative to the limbs. Data from the Quebec Family Study suggest that the size of the internal fat stores are more strongly influenced by genetic factors than subcutaneous fat depots[2]. Familial clustering analysis suggests that genetic factors may account for 37% of the variance in the trunk to extremity skinfold thickness ratio[8].

The combined evidence from these genetic analyses suggests that obesity is a polygenic disorder and that a considerable proportion of the variance is non-additive. This would explain the higher correlations between siblings than those between parent and offspring, and the 2-fold greater correlation between monozygotic than dizygotic twins. These genetic influences seem to operate through susceptibility genes; the occurrence of the gene increases the risk of developing a characteristic but is not essential for its expression nor is it, in itself, sufficient to explain the development of the disease.

Animal models of obesity   Animal models of obesity may derive from lesions in the ventro-medial hypothalamus, the paraventricular hypothalamus or the amygdala. Alternatively, there are autosomal recessive gene defects, of which the best known are *ob/ob* or *db/db* mice and *fa/fa* rats and a few less well-known polygenic models, such as the Japanese mouse. There are also models of dietary-induced obesity, which can be precipitated by feeding high carbohydrate diets (e.g. Spiny mouse), high fat diets (Osborne–Mendel rat) or cafeteria diets (e.g. Sprague–Dawley rat).

There is currently particular interest in the gene defect in the *ob/ob* mouse. This has been shown to be responsible for a failure to produce the hormone, leptin[9]. Injections of recombinant leptin lead to reductions in body weight, percent fat, serum glucose and insulin[10]. Injections into the lateral ventricle or third ventricle of the brain suggest there may be a central site of action, probably by reducing the concentration of neuropeptide-Y[11]. The leptin receptor has now also been cloned[12]. In man, the *ob* gene has 84% overall homology with that of the mouse but, in adipose tissue of obese subjects, *ob* mRNA is present at high levels and there are much higher serum concentrations of leptin in obese than normal weight humans[13,14]. It is possible that obese humans have a relative insensitivity to leptin or decreased transport into the CSF[15]. However, no structural or functional defects of the leptin-effector system in humans have yet been identified. The effects of the *ob* gene are mediated through effects on both energy intake and energy expenditure. The mice are hyperphagic and constantly search for food. They also have a defect in thermogenesis, mediated through the activity of the sympathetic nervous system and have low levels of spontaneous physical activity.

Candidate genes   Unlike animal models, where a number of single gene defects can lead to obesity, no human obesity gene has yet been characterised, but the heterogeneous nature of human obesity does not preclude the identification of small numbers of individuals with a single gene defect which leads to obesity. A number of so called candidate genes have been identified which are associated with the obese phenotype: these include the β_3 adrenergic receptor, lipoprotein lipase, dopamine receptor D_2, glucocorticoid receptor, TNF and apolipoprotein B, D and E genes[16].

In man, a number of genetically determined conditions result in excess body weight or fatness (e.g. Prader–Willi syndrome or Bardet–Biedl syndrome), but these cases account for only a very small proportion of the obese population.

Gene–environment interactions The susceptible gene hypothesis implies that environmental factors play a key role in unmasking latent genetic tendencies to develop obesity. This has been investigated in studies in which pairs of twins have been exposed to periods of positive and negative energy imbalance. Here, the within pair differences in the rate of weight gain, the proportion of weight gained as fat and the sites of fat deposition showed greater similarity than the between pair differences[17]. This suggests that differences in genetic susceptibility within a population may determine which individuals are most likely to become obese in any given set of environmental circumstances. These effects may be mediated by changing the individual's sensitivity to environmental exposures. Putative mechanisms for such effects may include altered sensitivity to gastrointestinal or neuro-peptides which control appetite and satiety, specific taste preferences, sympathetic nervous system (SNS) activity or differences in patterns of spontaneous physical activity. Studies of gene–environment interactions which may determine human obesity are complicated by the fact that the clinical features of obesity may be modulated over time and that there is a time-lag between environmental exposures, lifestyle choices and weight gain. There are also substantial inter-individual differences which need to be explained.

Physiological mediators

Energy expenditure

Studies in animals have suggested that during overfeeding a significant increase in metabolic rate may dissipate the excess energy thus reducing the rate of weight gain below theoretical values[18]. Genetically obese animals gain more weight than their lean controls even when they are pair-fed, implying a greater metabolic efficiency[19]. One possible mechanism for this effect is a decrease in diet-induced thermogenesis which is attenuated in animal models of obesity due to a decrease in the sympathetic activation of brown adipose tissue[20]. These unequivocal effects on energy expenditure in obese animals contrast with the paucity of evidence in humans. Nonetheless, in obese humans, there have been persistent reports of abnormally low energy intakes which indirectly imply that there must be a defect in energy expenditure. There are three principal components to energy expenditure which have each been the subject of detailed research.

Basal metabolic rate Basal or resting metabolic rate is the energy expended by an individual at rest, following an overnight fast and at a comfortable environmental temperature in the thermoneutral range. Numerous studies of basal metabolic rate have conclusively demonstrated that obese subjects have an increased BMR relative to their lean counterparts[21]. Figure 1 shows data from a recent analysis[22] of basal energy expenditure in 319 obese subjects in which the BMR of the women with a BMI less than 25 kg/m² is only 5.71 ± 0.54 MJ/day compared to 8.23 ± 1.21 MJ/day in those with a BMI > 35 kg/m². The increase in BMR is predominantly due to an increase in the fat-free mass which increases alongside fat mass.

Approximately 80% of the inter-individual variance in BMR can be accounted for by age, fat-free mass, fat mass and gender[23]. Nonetheless, this still leaves some potential for inter-individual differences in BMR which may predispose individuals with a relatively low BMR to become obese. Longitudinal studies of the Pima Indians suggest that the risk of gaining 10 kg in the subsequent 4 year follow up was 7-fold greater in those in the lowest tertile of relative BMR than those in the highest tertile[24]. However, it predicts only about 40% of the weight gain, and the increase in body weight is in itself still associated with an increase in resting metabolism which normalises BMR. Similar observations have also been made in infants and in children[25]. Putative mechanisms for these effects include differences in SNS activity or skeletal muscle metabolism. However, this is not a consistent predictor in other populations. For example Seidell *et al.* found no association between BMR and

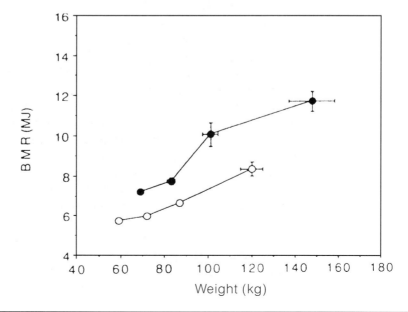

Fig. 1 Influence of body weight on basal metabolic rate in women (open circles) and men (closed circles) analysed by BMI category (< 25, 25.0–29.9, 30–34.9, > 35 kg/m²). Reproduced with permission from Prentice *et al.* [22]

10 year weight gain in 775 men and women[26] and others have also questioned the validity of this putative association.

Studies of resting energy expenditure in post-obese subjects matched to never-obese controls have usually found no difference in BMR, although a recent combined analysis of 11 published studies of energy expenditure in the post-obese concluded that there was a 5% decrease in resting energy expenditure, which would be too small to be statistically significant in many of the individual studies with small groups of subjects[27].

Diet-induced thermogenesis A number of studies have suggested that the post-prandial increase in energy expenditure is attenuated in obese subjects, perhaps due to decreased SNS activity (for example[28]). Similar effects have also been demonstrated in the post-obese. However, this is not a consistent finding, even among studies from the same laboratory. A recent review has identified 28 studies in favour of a defect in thermogenesis in humans and 17 against[29]. This variability may be due in part to methodological issues, since this is the least reproducible component of energy expenditure. However, since thermogenesis accounts for only a fraction of total energy expenditure (approximately 10%), the potential for a significant effect on total energy expenditure is small.

It has been suggested that the capacity for facultative thermogenesis may explain the differential propensity to weight gain during periods of overfeeding, a process described as luxus consumption. Although there was considerable support for this in the 1960s, the most recent studies, under carefully controlled conditions and with rigorous measurement techniques, do not suggest any significant role for this process in the modulation of energy balance during overfeeding[30,31]. It is imperative to make accurate measurements of changes in body composition during overfeeding, since differences in nutrient partitioning between lean and fat tissue will lead to differences in absolute weight gain for a similar energy excess because of the differences in the energy density of tissue gained. Data from the Minnesota study, in which 32 subjects were underfed for 24 weeks and then progressively re-fed, show that the proportion of weight gained as protein (p-ratio) during refeeding was strongly correlated with the p-ratio during weight loss[32]. Moreover, in a multiple regression analysis, the p-ratio was strongly correlated with the magnitude of the decrease in thermogenesis during weight loss.

Physical activity The most variable component of energy expenditure is physical activity which may represent 20–50% of total energy expenditure. Studies of fidgeting movements in Pima Indians within a whole-body calorimeter have shown significant inter-individual variations in the daily energy cost of these actions from 400–3000 kJ/day, with low levels predictive of subsequent weight gain at least in males but not females[33]. However, in free-living conditions, the freedom to undertake conscious physical activity or exercise increases the inter-individual variability even further.

Research in this area has been hampered by imprecision in the methods to measure physical activity which have included various actometers, heart rate monitoring, activity diaries and direct observation. However, a stable isotope technique, the doubly-labelled water method, allows accurate measurements of habitual total energy expenditure (TEE) over a 10–20 day period[34]. The ratio of TEE/BMR gives the physical activity level (PAL), an index of the physical activity of the subjects. When analysed in relation to BMI, the PAL is similar in groups of subjects with a BMI < 20, 20–25 and 25–35 kg/m^2 in both men and women, suggesting similar levels of habitual activity[22]. The PAL ratio is reduced in grossly obese subjects (BMI > 35 kg/m^2) where it seems reasonable to assume that their size becomes physically incapacitating. Although these measurements were made in subjects with established obesity, it is unlikely that they have become increasingly active as their weight has increased; so it appears that, during the dynamic phase of weight gain, there is little evidence that obese people were less active than their lean counterparts.

Total energy expenditure The energy requirements of an individual reflect the sum of basal expenditure, thermogenesis and physical activity. Total energy expenditure can be measured under experimental conditions using a whole-body calorimeter. Studies of age and sex matched pairs of lean and obese women clearly demonstrate that, whilst following an imposed activity schedule, the energy expenditure of obese subjects is consistently higher than their lean pair (Fig. 2)[35]. Energy expenditure measured at home during everyday activities using doubly-labelled water shows a similar elevation, although when corrected for differences in body size there is no significant difference between lean and obese women. The analysis of total energy expenditure in 319 obese subjects clearly demonstrates a significant increase in energy expenditure with increasing body weight such that individuals with a BMI in excess of 35 kg/m^2 have an energy expenditure approximately 30% higher than those with a BMI less than 25 kg/m^2 (Fig. 3)[22].

The outstanding difficulty with these studies is that the increase in energy expenditure seen in obese subjects as a consequence of their increased body size may conceal pre-existing metabolic defects in the pre-obese state which predisposed the individual to excessive weight gain. However, in experimental overfeeding studies, there is no significant difference in the rate of weight gain between lean and obese

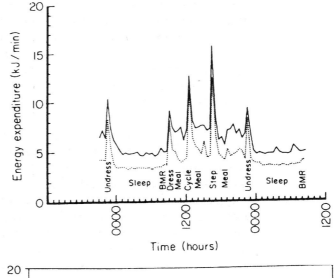

Fig. 2 Energy expenditure measured over 37 h in a whole-body calorimeter in lean (broken line) and obese women (solid line). Reproduced with permission from Prentice et al. [21]

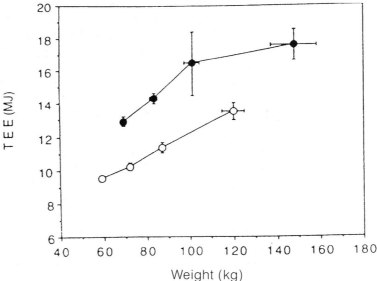

Fig. 3 Influence of body weight on total energy expenditure in women (open circles) and men (closed circles) analysed by BMI category (< 25, 25.0–29.9, 30–34.9, > 35 kg/m²). Reproduced with permission from Prentice et al. [22]

subjects when matched for their excess energy intake[30]. Studies of total energy expenditure in post-obese subjects have been less conclusive; some studies show no difference in energy expenditure in the post-obese relative to never-obese controls[36], whilst others show a modest suppression of energy expenditure[37]. However, the magnitude of the effect is small and may reflect either metabolic or behavioural differences between the groups.

Overall, there is little evidence to support the hypothesis that human obesity may be due to a specific defect in energy expenditure in predisposed individuals. However, advocates of a metabolic basis to obesity argue that only very small differences in energy expenditure are required to produce sustained weight gain over many years, and this difference may be below the limits of precision of even the most sophisticated methodology.

Substrate oxidation Energy balance can also be considered as the sum of individual macronutrient balances. For subjects in energy balance, the fuel oxidised will have a similar composition to that consumed. Thus, changes in the composition of the diet can have a profound influence on substrate oxidation in the absence of changes in total energy expenditure. Calorimetry studies, with constant diets, suggest that the modulation of substrate oxidation may take 3–5 days to re-establish macronutrient balance[38]. In free-living situations where the composition of day-to-day food intake is more variable, the previous day's diet composition exerts a strong influence on the subsequent day's substrate oxidation. This has the potential to produce artefactual results in studies in which antecedent diet is not carefully controlled.

Flatt has proposed that the positive fat balance associated with the aetiology of obesity reflects a failure to increase fat oxidation to match dietary fat intake[39]. In support of this hypothesis, Astrup *et al.* have demonstrated that post-obese subjects (who have previously demonstrated a predisposition to obesity) have an impaired ability to increase the rate of fat oxidation when challenged by a high fat diet[40–42]. They have suggested that the development of obesity may represent a mechanism to compensate for this defect and to facilitate increases in fat oxidation to match the amount of fat consumed. This may be achieved through higher circulating concentrations of non-esterified fatty acids and insulin resistance which favours fat oxidation. However, this would imply a self-limiting mechanism, which is clearly not always the case.

Longitudinal studies in the Pima Indian population have shown that subjects with a relatively high 24 hour respiratory quotient (RQ; reflecting a high ratio of carbohydrate to fat oxidation) are at 2.5 times the risk of gaining > 5 kg than those with a lower RQ[43]. Moreover, 28% of the variance in RQ can be explained on the basis of familial associations, which may partly explain the aggregation of obesity in families. In the Quebec Family Study, the heritability of RQ was assessed to be 20%[44]. Given the effects of antecedent diet on measured RQ, these similarities could have resulted from similar habitual diets. However, when diet was controlled within a 100 day overfeeding study in identical twins, the within-pair resemblance in RQ was greater than the between-pair effects[45].

The mechanism of a putative genetic determinant in fuel selection is unclear although there is evidence that it may be mediated via plasma concentrations of triiodothyronine (T$_3$) and androstenedione, SNS activity, or the activities of key enzymes in the β-oxidation pathway. It has also been hypothesised that skeletal muscle may be an important site of differences in fuel selection, either through the effects of insulin sensitivity or muscle fibre type. Type I muscle fibres have a higher capacity for substrate oxidation and thus a low ratio of Type I to Type II fibres may predispose to low fat oxidation and obesity. Wade found an inverse relationship between body fatness and the proportion of type 1 muscle fibres[46], but other studies have found no significant relationship[47] and have suggested that the link may be an artefact of different levels of physical fitness[48]. This remains an important area of research.

Energy intake

The failure to identify a defect in the metabolic control of energy expenditure, and the contrary observation of high levels of energy expenditure in obese subjects has led to a focus on food intake to explain the aetiology of obesity. The increase in energy expenditure associated with the development of obesity should automatically help to prevent continued weight gain, hence the failure of this auto-regulatory system suggests that there must be a considerable error in the regulation of food intake. Furthermore, habitually lean individuals are able to regulate intake to match energy requirements over a wide range of energy requirements yet those who become obese seem unable to achieve this balance.

Under-reporting of food intake   Progress in understanding the role of energy intake in the aetiology of obesity has been seriously confounded by the profound under-reporting which is now widely recognised as a feature of obesity. Comparisons of energy intake and energy expenditure show consistent shortfalls in self-reported intake, averaging approximately 30% of energy requirements in obese subjects[35,49]. This phenomenon also extends to post-obese subjects and to others who may be very weight conscious. Figure 4 shows the comparison of reported energy intake with measured energy expenditure for individual subjects. In the obese group, the mean under-reporting was −36% and in the post-obese group −27%[50].

There may be a number of causes of under-reporting. It is common for individuals to change their eating habits as a consequence of the pressure of recording their food intake. This is usually associated with a reduction

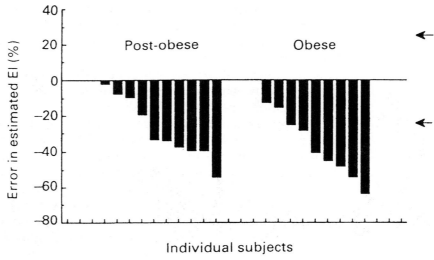

Fig. 4 Differences between self-reported energy intake and measured energy expenditure for post-obese and obese women. Arrows mark limits of measurement precision. Reproduced with permission from Jebb and Prentice[94].

in intake as subjects consciously or sub-consciously adopt a self-imposed 'diet'. Thus they may accurately report their intake for that week, but it is not representative of their habitual diet. Other causes of under-reporting may include forgetfulness, underestimation of portion size and inadequate knowledge of food composition. However, it is probable that there are also instances of self-deception or deliberate manipulation of dietary records. Under-reporting is such a reproducible bio-behavioural observation in obese people that it may in itself represent part of the aetiological syndrome of obesity through a failure to acknowledge true food intake.

Appetite control   Recent research into the appetite control system has identified a network of synchronous interactions which govern eating behaviour[51]. These effects are mediated through the central nervous system particularly the hypothalamus, where a number of neuropeptides appear to regulate feeding behaviour via effects on hunger and satiety. Laboratory studies of feeding behaviour have suggested that, following a covert energy preload, obese subjects may be less able to accurately compensate for the energy content of the preload at a subsequent meal than lean subjects[52]. However, these studies are usually of short duration in laboratory settings and may not accurately reflect eating behaviour in a naturalistic setting, where knowledge of foods consumed and conditioned learning may invoke other regulatory processes.

Macronutrient selection   There is abundant evidence that the individual macronutrients (protein, fat, carbohydrate and alcohol) exert different effects on eating behaviour, predominantly due to their effects on satiety[53]. Experimental studies of manipulated foods and retrospective analyses of dietary records suggest that protein is the most satiating[54,55]. Carbohydrate is also an efficient inhibitor of later food consumption, at least in the short term, meal-to-meal context[56]. A variety of carbohydrates suppress subsequent intake roughly in proportion to their energy content[57]. The evidence in relation to the effects of dietary fibre is less clear.

Fat appears to have a weak satiating capacity[58]. Subjects readily overeat in response to high fat foods[59]. This effect seems to occur within a single meal and has been described as high fat hyperphagia or passive overconsumption. However since fat has twice as much energy per gram as protein or carbohydrate, this may simply be a consequence of energy density and not a specific property of dietary fat *per se*[60]. Studies in which lean individuals were confined to a whole-body calorimeter for 7 days and allowed to eat *ad libitum* from a diet providing 20, 40 or 60% energy as fat, on three separate occasions, ate significantly more energy on the high fat diet and gained weight[61]. However, when the energy density of the three diets was constant, the high fat hyperphagia was abolished[62].

Alcohol has been claimed to have appetite stimulating effects. In free-living circumstances, alcohol consumption with meals is associated with higher energy intakes, but this may also reflect the fact that alcohol is more likely to be consumed on special occasions which in themselves are associated with increased food intake[63]. In experimental circumstances, a preload of alcohol has a similar effect to carbohydrate, suppressing subsequent intake and partially, but not completely, compensating for its energy content[64].

Sensory preferences The sensory perception of palatability may influence the amount and type of food consumed. This might be expected to exert its effects predominantly within a meal, by prolonging the duration of eating and quantity of a particular food consumed. Hence, sensory properties may have acute effects on energy intake and thus energy balance, but these effects may be rather more limited in the long term.

There have been numerous reports of sensory preferences for particular food groups in association with obesity, but inter-subject variability is so great as to obscure any underlying obese–lean differences[65]. Experimental studies of taste preferences have moved beyond classical taste tests to more complex food-like stimuli. Drewnowski has identified a relationship between the relative taste preference for fat versus sugar and BMI. Anorectic, low BMI women expressed a preference for foods with a high sugar to fat ratio and obese women the reverse, i.e. increasing overweight was associated with enhanced preference for fat[66]. Unfortunately, simple measures of liking for specific foods do not necessarily correspond to actual dietary intake behaviour. Dietary surveys reveal few, if any, relationships between specific food selections and relative body weight. In community-based studies, the inter-subject variability in preferences was greater than the obese–lean differences[67].

It is plausible to suggest that individuals predisposed to obesity may be hyper-sensitive to the hedonic properties of food (see externality). A recent study has demonstrated that post-diet weight regain in women was associated with preferences for high fat-high sugar desserts[68].

Eating frequency Some epidemiological studies have suggested that individuals who report eating a greater number of small meals have a lower relative weight than those eating fewer meals and it has been inferred that the consumption of large meals may be a risk factor for obesity. However, a recent review of the literature failed to find any significant association[69]. Research in this area is confounded by under-reporting of intake in obese subjects and by *post-hoc* changes in eating habits as a consequence of obesity and attempts at weight control. Measuring eating frequency in subjects with established obesity is an unreliable guide to the eating practices involved in its aetiology.

The putative mechanisms whereby frequent feeding episodes may modulate energy balance are unclear. Some studies[70] have suggested a higher thermic effect of food associated with 'gorging' relative to 'nibbling', but measurements made over a 24 h period to not support this hypothesis[71]. It is more likely that any effects are mediated through changes in appetite and hence energy intake. Studies of the effect of variation in feeding frequency during voluntary dieting have not observed any effect on the rate of weight loss[69].

Environmental factors

Environmental factors may play a critical role in the development of obesity by unmasking genetic or metabolic susceptibilities. Examples of this come from the Naura in Micronesia, and Polynesians in Western Samoa. There has been a dramatic change in diet and lifestyle in these communities over a very short period of time, resulting in an age standardised prevalence of obesity in men and women of 60% or more[72]. There are also a number of migrant studies, where populations with a common genetic heritage now live under very different environmental circumstances. Pima Indians living in the US average 25 kg heavier than comparable subjects living in Mexico[73]. A recent study of migrant

Africans living in the Caribbean or US showed a significant increase in the prevalence of obesity in comparison to their native countries of Nigeria or Cameroon[74]. In Nigeria, the mean BMI was 21.7 ± 3.6 kg/m^2 in men and 22.6 ± 4.7 kg/m^2 in women, whereas in the US, the average was 27.1 ± 5.5 kg/m^2 and 30.8 ± 7.7 kg/m^2, respectively. The increased prevalence of obesity is also associated with an increase in adverse health consequences, such as hypertension, which ranges from only about 15% in those living in Africa to over 30% among those in the US.

Environmental influences must act via an increase in energy intake and/or a decrease in energy expenditure and there is a substantial body of evidence which has investigated these effects both within and between populations. Cross-cultural dietary studies have failed to show a consistent relationship between nutritional factors and relative weight, although within populations there is some evidence that high fat diets are associated with an increased risk of obesity[75]. These studies are frequently confounded by under-reporting of dietary intake, which may be a particular problem if the bias is unevenly distributed across the different populations. To some extent, this can be minimised by considering the proportion of dietary energy derived from each macronutrient. For example, in the Scottish arm of the MONICA study, there is a positive association between the proportion of dietary fat and BMI and a negative association with the proportion of carbohydrate (particularly simple sugars), for both men and women[76]. When expressed as the fat to sugar ratio, there is a 3-fold difference in the prevalence of obesity in men and a 2-fold difference in women in the upper and lower quintiles of macronutrient intake. Although such studies have formed the basis of the hypothesis that dietary fat is an aetiological determinant of obesity, this has not been conclusively demonstrated by the more rigorous prospective studies. This may be due in part to the difficulties of making reliable estimates of energy and macronutrient intake. The metabolic evidence presented above, that dietary fat may undermine appetite regulation, continues to make this a plausible hypothesis.

Cross-cultural studies of physical activity and BMI, have shown that there is a 7-fold increased risk of overweight (BMI >25 kg/m^2) in those with a PAL ratio of <1.8 and within developed countries there is a relationship between low levels of physical activity and an increased likelihood of becoming obese[77]. In a large study in Finland ($n = 12,669$), those reporting physical exercise three or more times per week had, on average, lost weight since a preceding survey 5 years earlier, whilst those with little physical activity had gained weight and had twice the risk of gaining in excess of 5 kg than the physically active subjects[78]. Other studies have examined the relationship of obesity to sedentary behaviours *per se*, notably TV viewing (an almost invariably totally

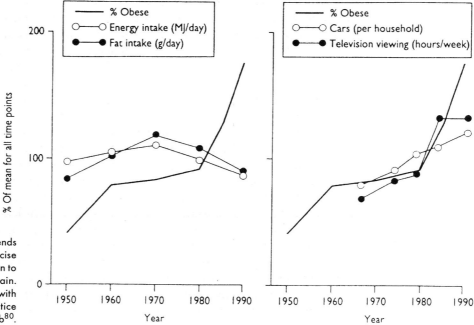

Fig. 5 Secular trends in diet (left) and exercise (right) in relation to obesity in Britain. Reproduced with permission from Prentice and Jebb[80].

inactive pursuit). Among children in the US, the relative risk of obesity was 5.3 times greater for children who watched more than 5 h TV per day compared with those who watched less than 2 h, even after correcting for a wide range of socio-economic variables[79].

In the UK, a study has combined data on energy intake and physical activity in relation to the secular increase in obesity in which the proportion of clinically obese subjects has increased from <2% in 1930 to 15% in 1994[80]. This shows that there has been no relationship between either total energy intake or fat consumption and the prevalence of clinical obesity over the last 60 years, whilst proxy measures of physical inactivity (TV viewing and car ownership) are closely related (Fig. 5). A study analysing trends in energy intake and expenditure in recent years, as part of the Finn Monica study suggests that these changes are now becoming less marked[81]. Between 1982 and 1992, the prevalence of obesity (BMI >27 kg/m^2) increased from 39% to 43% in men and 33% to 34% in women. During this time, energy intake declined in both groups but, when suspected under-reporters were excluded, the decrease was only 519 kJ/day in men and 347 kJ/day in women. Physical activity at work and in transport declined, although there was a significant increase in leisure time activity. Overall, the net energy cost of physical activity in women was unchanged and in men decreased by 3%. These data suggest that, in recent years, the **apparent** secular decrease in energy intake may be largely due to an increased prevalence of under-reporting and that increased leisure time activity may at least partially offset the decline in manual occupations.

In spite of the epidemiological evidence that environmental factors are playing an important role in the aetiology of obesity, it is a fact that within a population there are also a significant number of people who are able to control their weight. Analysis of the prevalence of obesity by socio-economic status shows a strong social class gradient, especially in women, in the UK ranging from 10.7% in social class I (high) to 25% in social class V (low)[82]. There is evidence that although the types of foods consumed across the social groups may be very different, total energy and fat intake is remarkably constant[80]. However, there are marked differences in measures of physical activity. UK national surveys show that those in social classes IV and V spend significantly more time watching TV and are more likely to define themselves as inactive compared to those in social class I. However, in a stepwise multiple regression analysis, the social class gradient in obesity in women persisted even after correction for physical activity and other lifestyle variables such as smoking and alcohol consumption[83]. This implies that there may be other individual factors which have not been considered that play an important role in modulating the risk of obesity, such as the cognitive control of food intake.

Psycho-social influences

Studies of the aetiology of human obesity are complicated by the potential for voluntary or cognitive factors to over-ride many physiological regulatory systems. Cultural factors operating through gender, ethnic, socio-economic or familial hierarchies provide a powerful determinant of body weight by setting moral and social connotations to body weight and defining attitudes to eating and exercise behaviours. Against this background, a number of specific individual characteristics may place individuals at increased risk of obesity.

Externality

The 'externality theory' of obesity was first described by Schacter to explain the observation that, relative to lean controls, eating behaviour in obese humans appeared to be more sensitive to external cues, such as the time of day, sight or smell of food or the presence of others, than to internal cues of hunger or satiety[84]. Subsequent research suggested that externality was closely related to dietary restraint, but recent studies using improved psychometric measures of externality have shown a correlation of externality with BMI, even after controlling for restraint[85]. The effects of palatability on food consumption have recently been explored in the context of this theory. In most experimental studies, preferred foods are consumed in greater quantities than less preferred foods, but the magnitude of this effect is greater in obese subjects[86]. It seems probable that multiple aspects of 'externality' require further analysis as potential contributors to obesity.

Restraint

There is suggestive, but inconclusive, evidence for the role of restrained eating in the aetiology of obesity. Studies of eating behaviour show that restrained eaters report more food cravings and binge eating[87]. One of the characteristic features of dietary restraint is a tendency towards disinhibited eating in particular circumstances. In experimental situations, intake at a test meal is inversely related to the energy content of a preload in unrestrained eaters but, paradoxically, restrained eaters show a positive relationship between the size of the preload and subsequent intake[88]. This disinhibition may be a cognitive effect; restrained eaters given the same preload on two separate occasions ate more after the preload was identified as high energy rather than low energy. This effect might suggest that restrained eaters may be more susceptible to the availability of highly palatable foods, which act as a stimulus for excess food consumption. However, it is also possible that a degree of cognitive dietary restraint is necessary in order to protect against overconsumption in an environment with an excess supply of affordable and palatable foods.

Psychological disturbances

A number of specific psychological syndromes have been identified in obese subjects, but whether these represent a cause or consequence of obesity is unclear. Evidence of improvements in emotional well-being following successful treatment are indicative that many emotional disorders are secondary to obesity[89].

Binge eating in association with obesity was first described in 1959, but it has only recently been classified as a specific disorder, occurring when an individual consumes objectively large amounts of food with subjective sensations of a loss of control, on at least two occasions per week for 6 months[90]. One epidemiological study has shown that in women presenting for treatment, the onset of binge eating preceded the onset of obesity or dieting[91]. Some studies have linked binge eating to emotional distress. There is evidence of a higher level of both personality disorders and depression in binge eaters but, in many cases, the eating disorder precedes the development of other co-morbidity.

Many other obese subjects do not fulfil the strict classification for binge eating but, nonetheless, report being more likely to overeat at times when they are in a negative emotional condition. This is the basis of Kaplan's psychosomatic theory of obesity which hypothesises that obesity may be the consequence of early childhood experiences in which food was continually associated with comfort. However, there is little evidence in support of this beyond clinical case histories and no convincing evidence of an association between obesity and any particular personality type.

Stress

There is some evidence that stress, and more specifically an individual's capacity to control their stress levels, may play a role in the aetiology of obesity. Some studies report that stress is associated with the consumption of high fat foods and a community based study has linked stress to weight gain[92]. Bjorntorp has proposed a metabolic basis to this theory, particularly in the modulation of abdominal obesity, through the effects of stress on the hypothalamic–pituitary–adrenal axis and cortisol overproduction[93].

Conclusions

Obesity is probably one of the most complex diseases in respect to its aetiology. At its simplest, obesity will only develop when energy intake exceeds energy expenditure over a prolonged period, but this overview conceals the multiple influences on energy intake and expenditure and ignores the potential for a genetic predisposition. Accordingly, there is unlikely to be a single unifying theory to explain the aetiological basis of obesity. However, a better understanding of the aetiological determinants in individual subjects will provide a basis for more rational interventions to both prevent and treat this recalcitrant public health problem.

References

1   Heber D. The endocrinology of obesity. In: Blackburn G (ed) *BS Kanders*. New York: Chapman 98–109
2   Bouchard C, Perusse L, Leblanc C, Tremblay A, Theriault G. Inheritance of the amount and distribution of human body fat. *Int J Obes* 1988; **12** :205–15
3   Friedlander Y, Kark J, Kaufmann N, Barry E, Stein Y. Familial aggregation of body mass index in ethnically diverse families in Jerusalem: the Jerusalem Lipid Research Clinic. *Int J Obes* 1988; **12**: 237-47
4   Stunkard A, Harris J, Pedersen N, McClearn G. The body mass index of twins who have been reared apart. *N Engl J Med* 1990; **322**: 1483–7
5   Allison D, Kaprio J, Korkeila M, Koskenvuo M, Neale M, Hayakawa K. The heritability of body mass index among an international sample of monozygotic twins reared apart. *Int J Obes* 1996; **20**: 501–6
6   Stunkard A, Sorensen T, Hanis C *et al*. An adoption study of human obesity. *N Engl J Med* 1986; **314**: 193–8
7   Vogler G, Sorensen T, Stunkard A, Srinivasan M, Rao D. Influences of genes and shared family environment on adult body mass index assessed in an adoption study by a comprehensive path model. *Int J Obes* 1995; **19**: 40–5
8   Rice T, Bouchard C, Perusse L, Rao D. Familial clustering of multiple measures of adiposity and fat distribution in the Quebec Family Study: a trivariate analysis of percent body fat, body mass index and trunk-to-extremity skinfold ratio. *Int J Obes* 1995; **19**: 902–8
9   Zhang Y, Proenca R, Maffei M, Barone M, Leopold L, Friedman J. Positional cloning of the mouse gene and its human homologue. *Nature* 1994; **372**: 425–32
10 Pellymounter M, Cullen M, Baker M *et al*. Effects of the obese gene product on body weight regulation in *ob/ob* mice. *Science* 1995; **269**: 540–2
11 Stephens T, Basinski M, Bristow P *et al*. The role of neuropeptide-Y in the anti-obesity action of the obese gene product. *Nature* 1995; **377**: 530–2
12 Tartaglia L, Dempski M, Weng X *et al*. Identification and expression cloning of a leptin receptor, OB-R. *Cell* 1995; **83**: 1263–71
13 Lonnqvist F, Arner P, Nordfors L, Schalling M. Overexpression of the obese (*ob*) gene in adipose tissue of human obese subjects. *Nature Med* 1995; **1**: 950–3
14 Considine R, Sinha M, Heiman M *et al*. Serum immunoreactive-leptin concentrations in normal-weight and obese humans. *N Engl J Med* 1996; **334**: 292–5
15 Caro J, Kollaczynnski J, Nyce M *et al*. Decreased cerebrospinal-fluid/serum leptin ratio in obesity: a possible mechanism for leptin resistance. *Lancet* 1996; **348**: 159–61
16 Beales P, Kopelman P. Obesity genes. *Clin Endocrinol* 1996; **45** (4): 373–8
17 Poehlman E, Tremblay A, Depres JP. Genotype-controlled changes in body composition and fat morphology following overfeeding in twins. *Am J Clin Nutr* 1986; **43**: 723–31
18 Rothwell N, Stock M. Luxus consumption, diet-induced thermogenesis and brown fat: the case in favour. *Clin Sci* 1983; **64**: 19–23
19 Thurby P, Trayhurn P. The role of thermoregulatory thermogenesis in the development of obesity in genetically obese (*ob/ob*) mice pair-fed with lean siblings. *Br J Nutr* 1979; **42**: 377–85
20 Rothwell N, Stock M. A role for brown adipose tissue in diet-induced thermogenesis. *Nature* 1979; **281**: 31–5
21 Prentice AM, Black AE, Murgatroyd PR, Goldberg GR, Coward WA. Metabolism or appetite: questions of energy balance with particular reference to obesity. *J Hum Nutr Diet* 1989; **2**: 95–104
22 Prentice AM, Black AE, Coward WA, Cole TJ. Energy expenditure in affluent societies: an analysis of 319 doubly-labelled water measurements. *Eur J Clin Nutr* 1996; **50**: 93–7
23 Swinburn B, Ravussin E. Energy and macronutrient metabolism. *Baillière's Clin Endocrinol Metab* 1994; **8**: 527–48
24 Ravussin E, Lillioja S, Knowler W *et al*. Reduced rate of energy expenditure as a risk factor for body weight gain. *N Engl J Med* 1988; **318**: 467–72

25 Roberts S. Abnormalities of energy expenditure and the development of obesity. *Obes Res* 1995; **3**: 155S–63S

26 Seidell J, Muller D, Sorkin J, Andres R. Fasting respiratory exchange ratio and resting metabolic rate as predictors of weight gain: The Baltimore Longitudinal Study on Ageing. *Int J Obes* 1992; **16**: 667–74

27 Astrup A. Obesity and metabolic efficiency. In: Chadwick D, Cardew G (eds) *The Origins and Consequences of Obesity*. Chichester: Wiley, 1996: 159–73

28 Astrup A, Andersen T, Henriksen O *et al*. Impaired glucose-induced thermogenesis in skeletal muscle in obesity. The role of the sympathoadrenal system. *Int J Obes* 1987; **11**: 51–66

29 Ravussin E, Swinburn B. Energy Metabolism. In: Stunkard A, Wadden T (eds) *Obesity: Theory and Therapy*. New York: Raven, 1993

30 Diaz E, Prentice AM, Goldberg GR, Murgatroyd PR, Coward WA. Metabolic response to experimental overfeeding in lean and overweight healthy volunteers. *Am J Clin Nutr* 1992; **56**: 641–55

31 Tataranni P, Larson D, Snitker S, Ravussin E. Thermal effect of food in humans: methods and results from use of a respiratory chamber. *Am J Clin Nutr* 1995; **61**: 1013–9

32 Dulloo A, Jacquet J, Grardier L. Autoregulation of body composition during weight recovery in human: the Minnesota experiment revisited. *Int J Obes* 1996; **20**: 393–405

33 Zurlo F, Ferraro R, Fontvielle A *et al*. Spontaneous physical activity and obesity: cross-sectional and longitudinal studies in Pima Indians. *Am J Physiol* 1992; **263**: E296–E300

34 Coward WA. The doubly-labelled water method: principles and practice. *Proc Nutr Soc* 1988; **47**: 209–18

35 Prentice AM, Black AE, Coward WA *et al*. High levels of energy expenditure in obese women. *BMJ* 1986; **292**: 983–7

36 Goldberg GR, Black AE, Prentice AM, Coward WA. No evidence of lower energy expenditure in post-obese women. *Proc Nutr Soc* 1991; **50**: 109A

37 Geissler C, Miller D, Shah M. The daily metabolic rate of the post-obese and the lean. *Am J Clin Nutr* 1987; **45**: 914–20

38 Astrup A, Buemann B, Toubro S, Raben A. Defects in substrate oxidation involved in the predisposition to obesity. *Proc Nutr Soc* 1996; **55**: 817–28

39 Flatt J. Importance of nutrient balance in body weight regulation. *Diabetes* 1988; **4**: 571–81

40 Astrup A, Buemann B, Christiansen N, Toubro S. Failure to increase lipid oxidation in response to increasing dietary fat content in formerly obese women. *Am J Physiol* 1994; **266**: E592–E599

41 Beumann B, Toubro S, Raben A, Astrup A. Substrate oxidation in post-obese women on 72-h high fat diet. A possible abnormal postprandial response. *Int J Obes* 1994; **18** (**Suppl. 2**): 97A

42 Raben A, Anderson H, Christiansen N, Madsen J, Holst J, Astrup A. Evidence for an abnormal postprandial response to a high fat mean in women predisposed to obesity. *Am J Physiol* 1994; **267**: E549–E559

43 Zurlo F, Lillioja S, Puente AE-D *et al*. Low ratio of fat to carbohydrate oxidation as predictor of weight gain: study of 24-h RQ. *Am J Physiol* 1990; **259**: E650–E657

44 Bouchard C, Deriaz O, Perusse L, Tremblay A. Genetics of energy expenditure in humans. In: Bouchard C (ed) *The Genetics of Obesity*. London: CRC Press, 1994: 135–45

45 Bouchard C, Tremblay A, Despres JP *et al*. The response to long term overfeeding in identical twins. *N Engl J Med* 1990; **322**: 1477–82

46 Wade A, Marbut M, Round J. Muscle fibre type and aetiology of obesity. *Lancet* 1990; **335**: 805–8

47 Simoneau J, Tremblay A, Thierault G, Bouchard C. Relationships between the metabolic profile of skeletal muscle and body fat gain in response to overfeeding. *Med Sci Sports Exercise* 1994; **5**: S159

48 Geerling B, Alles M, Murgatroyd P, Goldberg G, Harding M, Prentice A. Fatness in relation to substrate oxidation during exercise. *Int J Obes* 1994; **18**: 453–9

49 Lichtman S, Pisarska K, Berman E *et al*. Discrepancy between self-reported and actual caloric intake and exercise in obese subjects. *N Engl J Med* 1993; **327**: 1893–8

50 Black A, Prentice A, Goldberg G *et al*. Measurements of total energy expenditure provide insights into the validity of dietary measurements of energy intake. *J Am Diet Assoc* 1993; **93**: 572–9

51 Blundell J. Food intake and body weight regulation. In: Bouchard C, Bray G (eds) *Regulation of Body Weight. Biological and Behavioural Mechanisms*. Chichester: Wiley, 1996: 111–33

52 Spiegel T, Shrager E, Stellar E. Responses of lean and obese subjects to preloads, deprivation and palatablility. *Appetite* 1989; **13**: 45–69

53 Stubbs R. Macronutrient effects on appetite. *Int J Obes* 1995; **19** (**Suppl. 5**): S11–S19

54 DeCastro J. Macronutrient relationships with meal patterns and mood in the spontaneous feeding behaviour of humans. *Physiol Behav* 1987; **39**: 561–9

55 Hill A, Blundell J. Comparison of the action of macronutrients on the expression of appetite in lean and obese humans. *Ann NY Acad Sci* 1990; **597**: 529–31

56 Rolls B, Kim-Harris S, Fischmann M, Foltin R. Satiety after preloads with different amounts of fat and carbohydrate: implications for obesity. *Am J Clin Nutr* 1994; **60**: 476–87

57 Rogers P, Blundell J. Separating the actions of sweetness and calories: effects of saccharin and carbohydrates on hunger and food intake in human subjects. *Physiol Behav* 1989; **45**: 145–53

58 Lawton C, Burley V, Wales J, Blundell J. Dietary fat and appetite control in obese subjects: weak effects on satiation and satiety. *Int J Obes* 1993; **17**: 409–16

59 Blundell J, Burley V, Cotton J *et al*. The fat paradox: fat-induced satiety signals but overconsumption on high fat foods. *Int J Obes* 1995; **19**: 832–5

60 Poppitt S. Energy density of diets. *Int J Obes* 1995; **19** (**Suppl. 5**): S20–S26

61 Stubbs R, Harbron C, Murgatroyd P, Prentice AM. Covert manipulation of dietary fat and energy density: effect on substrate flux and food intake in men eating *ad libitum*. *Am J Clin Nutr* 1995; **62**: 316–29

62 Stubbs R, Harbron C, Prentice AM. Covert manipulation of the dietary fat to carbohydrate ratio of isoenergetically dense diets: effect on food intake in feeding men *ad libitum*. *Int J Obes* 1996; **20**: 651–60

63 DeCastro J, Orozco S. Moderate alcohol intake and spontaneous eating patterns of humans: evidence of unregulated supplementation. *Am J Clin Nutr* 1990; **52**: 246–53

64 Foltin R, Kelly T, Fischman M. Ethanol as an energy source in humans: comparison with dextrose-containing beverages. *Appetite* 1993; **20**: 95–110

65 Witherley S, Pangborn R, Stern J. Gustatory responses and eating duration of obese and lean adults. *Appetite* 1980; **1**: 53–8

66 Drewnowski A, Halmi K, Gibbs J *et al*. Taste and eating disorders. *Am J Clin Nutr* 1987; **46**: 442–50

67 Pangborn R. Individuality in responses to sensory stimuli. In: Solms J, Hall R (eds) *Criteria of Food Acceptance: How a Man Chooses what he Eats*. Zurich: Foster, 1981: 70–8

68 Drewnowski A, Holden-Wiltse J. Taste responses and food preferences in obese women: effects of weight cycling. *Int J Obes* 1992; **16**: 639–72

69 Bellisle F, McDevitt R, Prentice AM. Meal frequency and energy balance. *Br J Nutr* 1997; **77** (Suppl 1): S57–S70

70 Tai M, Castillo P, Pi-Sunyer X. Meal size and frequency: effect on the thermic effect of food. *Am J Clin Nutr* 1991; **54**: 783–7

71 Venne-Verboeket WV, Westerterp K, Kester A. Effect of the pattern of food intake on human energy metabolism. *Br J Nutr* 1993; **70**: 103–15

72 James W. The epidemiology of obesity. In: Chadwick D, Cardew G (eds) *The Origins and Consequences of Obesity*. Chichester: Wiley, 1996: 1–16

73 Ravussin E. Metabolic differences and the development of obesity. *Metabolism* 1995; **9** (**Suppl. 3**): 12–4

74 Wilks R, McFarlane-Anderson N, Bennett F *et al*. Obesity in peoples of the African diaspora. In: Chadwick D, Cardew G (eds) *The Origins and Consequences of Obesity*. Chichester: Wiley, 1996: 37–53

75 Lissner L, Heitmann B. Dietary fat and obesity: evidence from epidemiology. *Eur J Clin Nutr* 1995; **49**: 79–90

76 Bolton-Smith C, Woodward M. Dietary composition and fat to sugar ratios in relation to obesity. *Int J Obes* 1994; **18**: 820–8

77 Ferro-Luzzi A, Martino L. Obesity and physical activity. In: Chadwick D, Cardew G (eds) *The Origins and Consequences of Obesity*. Chichester: Wiley, 1996: 207–27

78 Rissanen A, Heliovaara M, Knekt P, Reunanen A, Aroma A. Determinants of weight gain and overweight in adult Finns. *Eur J Clin Nutr* 1991; **45**: 419–30

79 Gortmaker S, Must A, Sobel A, Peterson K, Colditz G, Dietz W. Television viewing as a cause of increasing obesity among children in the United States. *Arch Pediatr Adolesc Med* 1996; **150**: 356–62

80 Prentice AM, Jebb SA. Obesity in Britain: gluttony or sloth? *BMJ* 1995; **311**: 437–9

81 Fogelholm M, Mannisto S, Vartiainen E, Pietinen P. Determinants of energy balance and overweight in Finland 1982 and 1992. *Int J Obes* 1996; **20**: 1097–104

82 Bennett N, Dodd T, Flatley J, Freeth S, Bolling K. *Health Survey for England 1993*. London: HMSO, 1995

83 Jebb SA, Prentice AM, Cole TJ. Obesity and social class in women: effects of smoking, drinking and physical activity. *Proc Nutr Soc* 1997; **56** (1A): 159A

84 Schachter S. Some extraordinary facts about obese humans and rats. *Am Psychol* 1971; **26**: 129–44

85 Strien TV, Fritjers J, Bergers G, Defares P. On the relationship between emotional and external eating behaviour. *Addict Behav* 1995; **20**: 585–94

86 Spitzer L, Rodin J. Human eating behaviour: a critical review of studies in normal weight and overweight individuals. *Appetite* 1981; **2**: 293–329

87 Wardle J. Dietary restraint and binge eating. *Behav Anal Modif* 1980; **4**: 647–60

88 Polivy J. Perception of calories and regulation of intake in restrained and unrestrained subjects. *Addict Behav* 1976; **1**: 237–43

89 Smith D, Marcus M, Kaye W. Cognitive–behavioural treatment of obese binge-eaters. *Int J Eat Disord* 1992; **12**: 257–62

90 American Psychiatric Association. *Diagnostic and Statistical Manual of the American Psychiatric Association*, 3rd edn. Washington DC: American Psychiatric Association, 1994

91 Mussell M, Mitchell J, Weller C, Raymond N, Crow S, Crosby R. Onset of binge-eating, dieting, obesity and mood disorders among subjects seeking treatment for binge eating disorder. *Int J Eat Disord* 1995; **17**: 395–401

92 McCann B, Warnick G, Knopp R. Changes in plasma lipids and dietary intake accompanying shifts in perceived workload and stress. *Psychosom Med* 1990; **52**: 97–108

93 Bjorntorp P. Visceral obesity: a 'civilisation syndrome'. *Obes Res* 1993; **1**: 206–22

94 Jebb SA, Prentice AM. Is obesity an eating disorder? *Proc Nutr Soc* 1995; **54**: 721–8

Neurobiology

John Wilding, Peter Widdowson and **Gareth Williams**

Diabetes and Endocrinology Research Group, University of Liverpool, Liverpool, UK

The role of neuropeptide Y (NPY), leptin and 5-HT and other neurotransmitters implicated in the regulation of energy balance are only now being fully investigated. Little is known about how they may interact with each other in this complex process. In evolutionary terms, the availability of excess food, and the risk of obesity, is only a recent occurrence in humans. Man, and perhaps other species, may not have developed a specialised neurochemical system for adjusting food intake during obesity. Hence perturbation of a single system, such as hypothalamic NPY or leptin, is unlikely to be directly responsible for the development of most obesity. In contrast, periods of food deprivation and partial starvation have been common in the animal kingdom and the multitude of neurotransmitters implicated in energy balance are more likely to be directed towards increasing food consumption and conserving energy than reducing appetite and increasing thermogenesis in the presence of excess.

The last few years have witnessed rapid advances in the understanding of the fundamental mechanisms that regulate body weight and fat content. This progress will undoubtedly continue in the future, and it is hoped that this will be rewarded with the development of new drugs to treat obesity. At present, however, it is unclear whether NPY, leptin, or other apparently strong candidates will be the winner in the lucrative race for the ideal anti-obesity drug.

Correspondence to:
Dr John Wilding,
Diabetes and
Endocrinology Research
Group, University of
Liverpool,
Liverpool L69 3BX UK

Dysregulation of the central mechanisms that control energy balance is now recognised to play a major role in the development of obesity. At present, many novel centrally acting anti-obesity drugs are in pre-clinical development, and two such compounds have recently been licensed in Europe and the US, suggesting that we may be seeing a renaissance in therapeutics designed to reduce body weight. These drugs have two possible mechanisms of action: to reduce appetite and food intake; or to increase energy expenditure through thermogenesis. The neurophysiological processes controlling appetite and thermogenesis are complex, undoubtedly involving many neurotransmitter systems which may play either key or complementary roles. Any classification of these systems is inevitably artificial, but it is useful to consider the central factors involved in weight regulation separately from peripheral signals which indicate nutritional state (Fig. 1). Most of this work has been undertaken

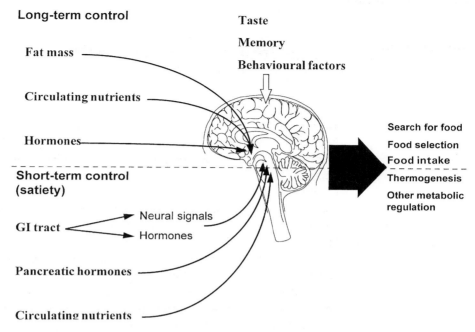

Fig. 1 Regulation of energy balance. Energy balance is regulated by the central nervous system, particularly the hypothalamus, which integrates signals indicating nutritional state, together with hedonic signals and memory of specific foods to control the type and

quantity of food eaten and the regulation of metabolism.

in rodents; it is likely that the same broad mechanisms apply to man, but the fine detail of the individual neurotransmitters and their physiological functions may differ considerably.

Central nervous system factors

Many substances have been suggested to play a role in body weight regulation (Table 1). This part of the review will mainly focus on two neurotransmitters, neuropeptide Y (NPY), which has recently attracted considerable attention, and the serotonin (5-HT) system, which is a major target for existing and future anti-obesity agents.

NPY is a 36 amino acid peptide which has emerged over the past 10 years as a possible key neurotransmitter candidate for the regulation of energy homeostasis. NPY is synthesised throughout the brains of rodents and humans, but is particularly abundant in the hypothalamus, a region crucial to the regulation of appetite[1]. Within the hypothalamus, NPY is synthesised largely in neurones whose cell bodies lie in the arcuate nucleus and which sends projections into surrounding hypothalamic structures, notably the paraventricular nucleus, where NPY is released from nerve terminals. Other NPY-containing neuronal projections that

Table 1 Neurotransmitters affecting food intake. A large number of neurotransmitters influence food intake; most are inhibitory. In general, neurotransmitters such as NPY, which increase food intake, also inhibit thermogenesis, and *vice versa*

Factors which increase food intake	Factors which inhibit food intake
Noradrenaline	Serotonin
Opioids	Dopamine
Growth hormone–releasing hormone	Cholecystokinin
Galanin	Corticotrophin–releasing factor
Neuropeptide Y	Neurotensin
Melanin–concentrating hormone	Bombesin
	Calcitonin gene–related peptide
	Amylin
	Adrenomedullin
	Glucagon
	Glucagon–like peptide–1

innervate hypothalamic structures originate from neurones situated in the medulla oblongata which cosynthesize catecholamines (Fig. 2).

Injections of NPY either into the cerebral ventricles or directly into specific hypothalamic regions, perhaps mimicking release of endogenous NPY, produces a potent and sustained increase in food intake within 10–15 min, combined with a reduction in thermogenesis[1]. Repeated injections of NPY into the brain over a few days result in obesity which is due to reduced thermogenesis and increased food intake[2], compounded by hyperinsulinaemia (see below). NPY is unique amongst neurotransmitters that increase food intake in that the NPY-induced hyperphagia does not become attenuated over time. Neuroanatomical mapping studies, using microinjection of NPY into discrete hypothalamic structures, have identified the paraventricular and perifornical

Fig. 2 Anatomy of the hypothalamus. This figure shows a schematic coronal section through the rat hypothalamus. The LH (lateral hypothalamus) and VMH (ventromedial hypothalamus) have traditionally been regarded as the feeding centre and the satiety centre respectively. This simplistic view is now outdated and the arcuate (ARC) and paraventricular (PVN) nuclei are now thought to be equally important.

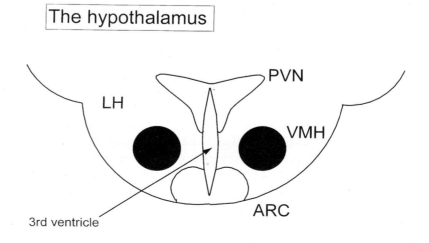

lateral hypothalamus as the areas most sensitive to the hyperphagic actions of NPY[3]. NPY inhibits thermogenesis by reducing the firing rate of sympathetic nerves which innervate brown adipose tissue in rodents. In addition to the hyperphagic actions of NPY and its ability to inhibit thermogenesis, direct injection of NPY into the hypothalamus also increases pancreatic insulin secretion, probably via the vagus. All these actions are consistent with a shift towards positive energy balance, stimulating energy intake and storing excess calories primarily as fat through the lipogenic actions of insulin[4].

There is now a large body of evidence demonstrating that hypothalamic NPY neurones become activated during conditions of negative energy balance, suggesting that an important role of NPY in the hypothalamus is to restore body energy stores. For example, NPY concentrations are elevated during starvation, food restriction and insulin-deficient diabetes in many hypothalamic structures innervated by the arcuate NPY neurones, most notably in the paraventricular nucleus. Synthesis in the arcuate nucleus (measured by mRNA levels) is also increased[1]. Blockade of endogenous NPY by infusion of monoclonal antibodies into the third ventricle reduces food intake when starved rats are refed, supporting a physiological role for NPY in the compensatory hyperphagia seen in conditions of negative energy balance[5].

NPY in obesity

Theoretically, inappropriate overactivity of the arcuate NPY neurones would lead to obesity, and there is convincing evidence that this is the case in certain instances. Most of the evidence indicating that increased hypothalamic NPY activity occurs in obesity has been generated using the genetically obese rodents, such as the fatty (fa/fa) Zucker rat and the ob/ob mouse[6,7]. The fatty Zucker rat is a model of severe obesity, which is characterized by hyperphagia, reduced brown adipose tissue thermogenesis and increased plasma insulin concentrations[6]. In this model, increased hypothalamic NPY activity has been demonstrated and may be responsible, in part, for the development of obesity[1,6]. Concentrations of NPY are increased in the arcuate and paraventricular nuclei and the levels of NPY mRNA are increased in the arcuate nucleus[6]. Furthermore, using push–pull cannulae to measure local NPY release, a sustained elevation in NPY release in and around the paraventricular nucleus is observed in the obese Zucker rat[8]. Finally, a reduction in NPY receptor numbers, consistent with downregulation, has been measured in whole hypothalamic blocks and in discrete hypothalamic structures, using quantitative receptor autoradiography, suggesting that there is a sustained and marked elevation in NPY release within the hypothalamus, particularly in regions supplied by the arcuate NPY neurones[9].

There have, however, been few attempts to investigate whether NPY is involved in the development of obesity in normal rats presented with highly palatable, high-energy foods, so-called 'cafeteria feeding'. This model is of particular importance as it is much closer to human obesity than the genetic syndromes. In one study, rats fed a palatable diet developed moderate obesity over 8 weeks; NPY concentrations were significantly elevated in the paraventricular, arcuate, medial preoptic and anterior hypothalamic nuclei in much the same way as in the Zucker rat. In contrast, however, there was no increase in total hypothalamic mRNA[10]. These results have been interpreted to indicate decreased, rather than increased NPYergic activity in diet-induced obesity, with the accumulation of unreleased NPY in nerve terminals to account for increased NPY concentrations in the sites of projection of the arcuate neurones. Further studies of the effect of diet-induced obesity on NPY release and NPY receptor density are required to assess the peptide's possible role in facilitating or acting against the development of obesity under these circumstances and their adaptive changes in states of positive energy balance.

NPY receptors and the NPY feeding receptor

Experiments using C-terminal fragments of NPY and substituted amino acids in the NPY sequence have demonstrated that NPY increases food intake through its interaction with a unique NPY receptor that is pharmacologically different from other known NPY receptors[11]. The first distinction between different NPY receptor subtypes was inferred when it was observed that C-terminal NPY fragments such as NPY_{13-36} were able to prejunctionally inhibit evoked contractions of the rat vas deferens. In contrast, post-synaptic actions, such as smooth muscle contraction, required the entire molecule. Pre-synaptic NPY receptors, sensitive to NPY_{13-36} are classified as Y_2-type receptors while post-synaptic NPY receptors are designated Y_1-type NPY receptors[11]. The C-terminally modified selective NPY Y_1 agonist, [Leu_{31}, Pro_{34}] NPY, but not NPY_{13-36}, stimulates feeding, suggesting that the receptor type responsible for the hyperphagia was more closely related to the Y1 subtype[12]. The NPY fragment, NPY_{2-36}, which is at least 10 times less potent than NPY in most Y_1 preparations is at least as equipotent as NPY in stimulating feeding, suggesting that the NPY feeding receptor must be pharmacologically distinct from Y1 receptors. Further experiments using NPY analogues have demonstrated two further

NPY receptors called Y3 and Y4. However, neither of these two new NPY receptors have the required pharmacological specificity of the NPY feeding receptor.

Recently, and nearly 5 years after the first suggestion that a unique NPY receptor mediated the feeding response, a novel NPY receptor was cloned from rat hypothalamus whose pharmacological properties matched with those expected of the NPY feeding receptor[13]. *In situ* hybridisation demonstrated that this 'Y5' receptor was expressed only in the brain and located largely to neuroanatomical structures associated with feeding, including the hypothalamic paraventricular, ventromedial and arcuate nucleii, the centromedial and reuniens thalamic nuclei, and some regions of the amygdala including the centromedial nucleus. Some brain regions expressed the Y5 receptor mRNA that were not closely associated with the control of food intake, notably the cerebral cortex, dentate gyrus and pyramidal CA3 region of the hippocampus[13]. Subsequently, a second group also cloned the Y5 receptor but this protein was 11 amino acids shorter at the N-terminus, suggesting that splice variants of the Y5 receptor gene may occur in rodent brains[14].

To complicate matters further, another novel NPY receptor was discovered in mouse hypothalamus (confusingly also termed 'Y5'), which had a substantially different amino acid sequence to the previously-reported Y5 receptor, but which displayed the required pharmacological profile of the feeding receptor, including high affinity for NPY, [Leu$_{31}$, Pro$_{34}$] NPY and NPY$_{2-36}$ but lower affinity for NPY$_{13-36}$[15]. This new NPY 'feeding' receptor was also expressed in different mouse brain regions to the receptors reported earlier, with high levels of expression in the paraventricular, anterior and preoptic hypothalamic nuclei[15].

Work is now underway to identify selective Y5 antagonists, which should clarify the role of the Y5 receptor in the regulation of food intake, and may ultimately be of therapeutic use in treating human obesity.

5-Hydroxytryptamine

The monamine neurotransmitters which include noradrenaline, adrenaline, dopamine and 5-hydroxytryptamine (5-HT, serotonin) have long been known to alter food intake in rodents, altering the quantity of food intake, the pattern of eating and appetite for specific nutrients. In contrast to noradrenaline and adrenaline, which stimulate food intake following intrahypothalamic injections, 5-HT suppresses food intake in freely-feeding or food-deprived rats. Using microinjections of 5-HT in various brain regions, its inhibitory actions on food intake have been localised to the hypothalamic paraventricular nucleus—the site at which NPY is most active in inducing feeding behaviour — and also in the ventromedial hypothalamus[16].

Pharmacological analysis of the 5-HT induced reduction in food intake has demonstrated that the effect is mediated by post-synaptic 5-HT_{1B} receptors[17]. In rats, selective 5-HT reuptake blocking drugs, (e.g. fluoxetine) are effective in reducing food intake, as are amphetamine-like drugs that both block 5-HT reuptake and stimulate 5-HT release, such as fenfluramine. In rats, fenfluramine virtually abolishes feeding over the first 4 h of darkness (when most food is consumed) demonstrating the potent effects of endogenous 5-HT to modulate food intake. In humans, however, the ability of drugs to elevate synaptic concentrations of 5-HT does not necessarily predict the ability to reduce appetite. Although D-fenfluramine is an effective anti-obesity drug, in at least a proportion of cases, fluoxetine and the selective 5-HT reuptake inhibitors, such as paroxetine and sertraline, do not reduce body weight (although high doses of fluoxetine have been clearly demonstrated to be effective in reducing bingeing in bulimic patients).

Recently, it has been suggested that elevations in both 5-HT and noradrenaline are required for the reduction in food intake in humans. A monoamine reuptake inhibitor drug called sibutramine, originally developed as an antidepressant, elevates both 5-HT and noradrenaline concentrations and potently inhibits feeding in rodents. Sibutramine has recently been submitted for registration in the US as a anti-obesity agent and its potential usefulness in humans is currently being explored in clinical trials[18].

5-HT and NPY interactions

Recent evidence suggests that the hypophagic actions of 5-HT may be mediated, at least partly, through the NPY pathway. For example, methysergide, a 5-HT antagonist which stimulates feeding, increases NPY concentrations in the arcuate and paraventricular nuclei of the hypothalamus[19]. Similarly, inhibition of 5-HT synthesis in the hypothalamus using p-chlorophenylalanine injected into the third ventricle also results in hyperphagia, and also produces an increase in NPY neuronal activity. Opposing these effects, m-chlorophenylpiperazine (mCPP), a 5-HT_1 agonist which reduces food intake, significantly reduces NPY concentrations in the hypothalamic paraventricular nucleus[20]. In addition, fenfluramine injections, which reduce food intake by raising synaptic concentrations of 5-HT, reduce concentrations of NPY in the dorsomedial, ventromedial and lateral hypothalamic nucleus[21]. The actions of fenfluramine on NPY activity and feeding appear complex, however, since NPY concentrations in the hypothalamic paraventricular and arcuate nuclei were not altered following an acute injection of fenfluramine, nor was the release of NPY from the paraventricular nucleus. Furthermore, D-fenfluramine did not alter NPY mRNA levels or regional NPY concentrations in a model of dietary obesity, despite producing weight loss[22]. Overall, these data suggest that NPY and 5-HT have opposing effects in the hypothalamus and that 5-HT may produce its hypophagic activity by directly inhibiting the firing of NPYergic neurones in the arcuate nucleus leading to reduced NPY release from the paraventricular nucleus. Fenfluramine appears to have a more complex mechanism of action, modulating the 5-HT and NPY neurones involved in feeding by altering the activity of medullary NPYergic projections to the lateral area, dorsomedial and ventromedial nuclei of the hypothalamus.

Corticotrophin-releasing factor (CRF) and glucagon-like peptide-1 (GLP-1)

CRF is expressed in the paraventricular nucleus and is an important regulator of ACTH secretion. CRF injected into the PVN causes weight loss, by reducing appetite and stimulating thermogenesis. It has been suggested that CRF and NPY act as opposing influences on the regulation of energy balance. CRF mRNA levels are altered in the opposite direction to NPY in conditions of energy deficit, such as food-deprivation and insulin-deficient diabetes. Furthermore, there is evidence of synaptic connections between CRF and NPY neurones in the paraventricular nucleus[23]. CRF may also interact with serotonin, as serotoninergic drugs, such as fenfluramine, decrease hypothalamic CRF concentrations[24].

The gut peptide GLP-1, an incretin hormone, is also synthesised within the rat brain and is effective at reducing food intake when injected into the third ventricle in the rat, both after food deprivation and after intracerebroventricular NPY injection. GLP-1 receptors are present in appetite regulating areas of the CNS, such as the paraventricular nucleus of the hypothalamus and the central nucleus of the amygdala. Injection of exendin 9–39, a selective GLP-1 antagonist, increases food intake in the rat and potentiates the appetite stimulating effect of NPY. GLP-1 is ineffective when given peripherally. Taken as a whole, these data suggest that GLP-1 may also play a role in the central component of the satiety sequence[25].

Peripheral signals

Peripheral signals involved in the regulation of body weight fall into two main groups. The first is the group of substances whose circulating concentrations rise after a meal, and are proposed as 'meal termination' or satiety signals. These may act on receptors in the periphery (for example on the vagus nerve) and transmit signals to the brain stem and other parts of the central nervous system, or act directly on the brain at sites where there is specialised modification of the blood–brain barrier, for example specific areas of the brain stem and hypothalamus. In addition to these humoral signals, there are direct neural signals which are initiated by phenomena such as stretching of the stomach wall and chemical signals originating within the gut.

The second group of substances are more concerned with long-term body weight regulation, and include hormones such as leptin, insulin and glucocorticoids, as well as levels of nutrients such as fatty acids and amino acids. It should be noted that some of these factors (such as insulin) may have dual role.

Satiety signals

Cholecystokinin (CCK)

CCK is the archetypal satiety signal. Its role in signalling satiety was suggested over 20 years ago[26], and there is now a considerable body of evidence supporting a physiological role for CCK as a meal termination signal. CCK is synthesised within the gut wall and is released into the portal circulation in response to the presence of nutrients (particularly fatty acids) within the gut. Further actions include stimulation of gall bladder contraction (hence its name) and pancreatic exocrine secretion. In rats, CCK injected either peripherally or into the central nervous system reduces food intake. This effect of peripheral CCK injection can be blocked by vagotomy[27].

CCK is now known to act via two different receptors, the CCK-A receptor and the CCK-B receptor (which is identical to the gastrin receptor), which are found both in the gastrointestinal tract and the central nervous system[28]. The development of specific antagonists of these receptors has allowed some clarification of the role of CCK in the regulation of food intake. Blockade of CCK-A receptors increases food intake by delaying the onset of satiety in rats, an effect thought to be predominantly mediated by inhibition of peripheral CCK-A receptors. Administration of CCK-B receptor antagonists blocks the effect of peripheral and centrally administered CCK and also increases food intake[29]. CCK stimulates receptors on the vagus nerve, which passes signals to the brain stem (probably the area postrema) and thus to other appetite-regulating areas, such as the hypothalamic paraventricular nucleus, where CCK appears to act as a neurotransmitter. It also seems likely that both receptors are involved, although the relative importance of the two subtypes at central and peripheral sites remains to be clarified.

There is some evidence that CCK also plays a physiological role controlling meal size in humans, based on careful infusion studies which mimic peripheral CCK concentrations after a meal[30]; on the other hand the CCK-A antagonist loxiglumide has so far failed to demonstrate an effect[31,32]. There are no reported studies of CCK-B antagonists in human satiety.

Glucagon and bombesin

A number of other 'gut-related' peptides have also been proposed as satiety factors. These include pancreatic glucagon and bombesin. There is presently little evidence for a role of these factors in humans, but bombesin reduces satiety in both humans and rodents when injected to mimic physiological concentrations[33,34]. Unlike CCK, this effect is not blocked by vagotomy, but can be blocked by vagotomy combined with disconnection of the sympathetic nerve supply to the gut[35]. Furthermore, food intake is increased when a specific bombesin antagonist is administered[36]. The evidence for native glucagon is less strong, and further research is needed in this area.

Long-term regulators of body weight

Although current interest is focused on leptin, other important factors are almost certainly involved in long-term weight regulation.

Insulin

Acute insulin administration causes hypoglycaemia, which produces hunger as one of its symptoms; the suggestion that insulin may act as a long-term satiety factor that reduces food intake may, therefore, seem surprising.

The ability of insulin to reduce weight was first observed in baboons infused insulin chronically into the cerebral ventricles[37]. Insulin antibodies administered intracerebroventricularly tend to increase body weight, supporting a physiological role for insulin in weight regulation[38,39]. Insulin receptors have been found within the central nervous system (particularly in the arcuate nucleus of the hypothalamus), but there is little evidence that insulin is synthesised within the CNS, and it seems more likely that circulating insulin is actively transported into the CNS[40].

Insulin, like leptin, may act in part by modulating the activity of NPY neurones in the arcuate nucleus. Insulin receptors are co-localized with NPY expression in the arcuate nucleus, and insulin administered ICV (albeit in high dose), is able to prevent or attenuate the rise in NPY mRNA seen in that nucleus during fasting[41].

Glucocorticoids

Clinically, it is well recognised that extremes of glucocorticoid production affect body fat and weight: excess glucocorticoids tend to produce truncal obesity (Cushing's syndrome) while deficiency results in weight loss (Addison's disease). However, it has been more difficult to establish a role for glucocorticoids in the normal regulation of body weight.

There is no doubt that corticosterone, the rodent counterpart of cortisol, is a necessary factor for the development of obesity in many rodent models of obesity. For example, adrenalectomy prevents weight gain in the *ob/ob* mouse and the Zucker rat[42,43]. Adrenalectomy is also effective in obesity caused by lesions of the ventromedial hypothalamus or by toxins such as gold thioglucose, an effect which can be reversed by intracerebroventricular, as well as systemic steroid replacement[44]. Adrenalectomy also attenuates the efficacy of many powerful appetite-stimulating agents, such as NPY[45]. The mechanisms by which glucocorticoids increase appetite is uncertain, but there are at least two strong possibilities which are not mutually incompatible. The first is the role of glucocorticoids in suppressing corticotrophin releasing factor (CRF), itself a powerful inhibitor of appetite. The second is via stimulation of NPY synthesis[46]. However, it is important to point out that the stimulatory effects of glucocorticoids on appetite in rodents and man are relatively weak, and as the strongest evidence for a role comes from studies looking at their absence, it may be better to consider them a necessary permissive agent for other factors such as NPY, rather than a direct regulator of appetite.

Leptin

The recent discovery of the fat-derived hormone called leptin (from the Greek *Leptos* meaning 'thin') has excited a great deal of academic and commercial interest. It has been proposed that leptin may be the long sought-after 'lipostat' factor postulated to govern energy balance through a negative feedback loop originating in adipose tissue and acting on centres in the brain[47]. This concept was supported by the work of Coleman whose elegant parabiosis experiments accurately predicted that the genetically-obese *ob/ob* mouse was lacking this lipostatic factor, while the *db/db* mouse was unable to respond to it, suggesting a defect in the receptor for the factor (Fig. 3)[48]. However, the mechanisms whereby fat-containing cells communicated to the brain was unknown[47]. The breakthrough occurred in 1994 through work aiming to identify the mutation responsible for producing obesity in the *ob/ob* mouse. Homozygosity for the *ob* (obese) gene results in reduced BAT activity and energy expenditure, hyperphagia and hyperinsulinaemia, which conspire to produce obesity as in the *fa/fa* Zucker rat. Using a positional cloning approach, the *ob* mutation was located within a gene encoding the 167-amino acid protein of 16 kDa, now known as leptin[49]. Leptin is expressed only in fat, and is secreted into the circulation. When injected into *ob/ob* mice, which do not produce functional leptin, food intake is markedly suppressed and body fat content falls without any reduction in

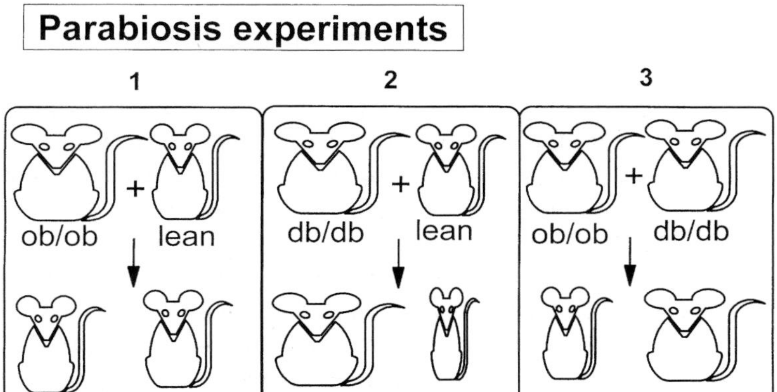

Parabiosis experiments

Fig. 3 Parabiosis experiments in lean, *ob/ob* and *db/db* mice. (1) When the circulation of an *ob/ob* mouse and a lean mouse are joined, the *ob/ob* mouse loses weight, suggesting that the *ob/ob* mouse is lacking a factor which causes weight loss. (2) If a *db/db* and a normal mouse are joined, the normal mouse loses weight, suggesting overproduction of a factor in the *db/db* mouse. (3) When a *db/db* and *ob/ob* mouse are joined, the *ob/ob* mouse again loses weight. Taken together these results support the hypothesis that the *ob/ob* mouse is lacking a weight regulating factor (now known to be leptin) and the *db/db* mouse its receptor.

lean body mass[50,51]. This selective loss of body fat is due to increased energy expenditure as well as hyperphagia, as the effect was greater with leptin than in untreated mice which were underfed to a comparable degree[50]. Leptin has similar effects in normal mice, but the effect is less marked; *db/db* mice (now known to have a leptin receptor defect) are unresponsive to exogenous leptin, as predicted from the parabiosis experiments.

Leptin receptors and transporters

Using autoradiography and *in situ* hybridisation techniques, leptin binding sites now known to correspond to various classes of leptin receptor have been identified in the hypothalamus, predominantly in the ventromedial and arcuate nuclei and the choroid plexus[52]. Leptin enters the brain intact via a saturable, active transport system that is independent from the insulin transporter[53]. This system effectively transports leptin across the blood brain barrier in the median eminence, one of the circumventricular organs, where specialised transport occurs between the circulation and the CNS. It has also been suggested that the high density of ^{125}I leptin binding sites in the choroid plexus and leptomeninges may also represent leptin transporters in these regions[52,54]. A single gene is now known to encode the various leptin receptor (Ob-R) isoforms in the brain and other tissues[55]. The leptin receptor is a single chain polypeptide with homology to cytokine receptors. It exists in two forms, with the same extracellular domain which binds leptin, but with differing intracellular regions. The short form (Ob-Ra) has a 34 amino acid intracellular portion and is thought to be the transporter, the long form (Ob-Rb) has a 304 amino acid intracellular domain which is probably responsible for intracellular signalling[52,55,56]. A number of other short leptin transporter isoforms have been reported, called Ob-Rc, Ob-Rd and Ob-Re, which are formed by alternative splicing of the leptin receptor gene in the rat[57]. Suggested functions for the short isoforms include the leptin transporter (Ob-Ra is expressed in the choroid plexus) and a circulating leptin transport protein (Ob-Re). As predicted by Coleman's experiments, defects in the leptin receptor also lead to obesity. Both *db/db* mice and *fa/fa* rats are phenotypically similar to *ob/ob* mice with obesity, hyperphagia, hyperinsulinaemia and reduced thermogenesis. The *db/db* mouse has a mutation that greatly truncates the intracellular portion of the receptor protein, so that all the isoforms terminate just inside the cell membrane[57]. By contrast, the *fa/fa* Zucker rat has a single point mutation (Gln to Pro) at amino acid 269 in the extracellular domain; the isoforms are, therefore, the correct length and the mutation has been suggested to interfere with the normal receptor dimerisation step which is thought to be necessary for the activated receptor to signal to the cell interior[58]. Like the related cytokine receptors, leptin receptor activity appears to depend on the activation of specific tyrosine kinases which phosphorylate further proteins in a cascade of events leading to alterations in gene activity[59]. In particular, the JAK-2 (Janus kinase-2), STAT-3 (STAT=signal transducers and activators of transcription), STAT-5 and STAT-6 kinases have all been implicated in the signalling process that follows binding of leptin to its receptor[59]. Taken together, these mutant rodent species demonstrate that a failure to produce sufficient leptin or a disturbance in the ability of the brain to respond to leptin, will result in obesity. As yet, however, no mutations in the gene encoding leptin or its transporter and receptor have been discovered in obese humans akin to the *db/db*, *ob/ob* or *fa/fa* mutations.

Leptin – NPY interactions

The actions of leptin in suppressing food intake and stimulating thermogenesis are apparently mediated in part by inhibiting NPY neurones in the hypothalamus[60]. Leptin may affect NPY neuronal activity at two separate sites. Leptin appears to reduce levels of NPY mRNA in the arcuate, and NPY levels in the ARC, PVN and MPO, implying concomitant inhibition of synthesis and transport (Fig. 4) [60,61]. Leptin may also have postsynaptic effects, reducing the activity of released NPY in that the hyperphagia induced by injections of NPY into the hypothalamus is attenuated by leptin administration. Interestingly, the transgenic NPY knockout-*ob/ob* mouse hybrid is halfway between normal lean and *ob/ob* mice in body weight, fat mass and other characteristics, supporting a role for NPY in mediating leptin action. This also suggests that there is at least one other major system involved in regulation of body weight in this model as suggested by normal food intake in NPY knockout mice[62].

Regulation of leptin production and secretion

Factors that determine leptin synthesis and release have now been studied in detail in rodents and some basic information about leptin in humans is now emerging. In rodents, it appears that the average daily circulating concentrations of leptin are related to body fat mass[63]. In addition, leptin secretion from fat is determined by hormonal status. Insulin and glucocorticoids increase leptin synthesis and secretion in rats,

Regulation of energy balance

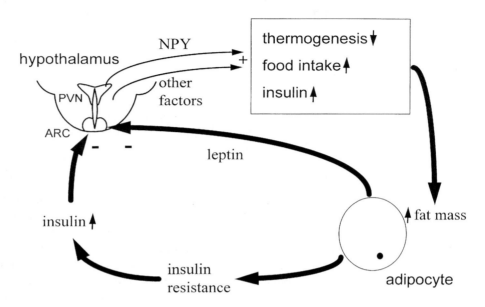

Fig. 4 Interactions between leptin, insulin and hypothalamic NPY. Leptin and insulin both have a negative influence on hypothalamic NPY and possibly other neurotransmitters involved in energy balance. If these effects are attenuated for any reason (extreme examples include leptin deficiency and leptin receptor mutations) then hypothalamic NPY synthesis and release increase, causing an increase in body weight via increased food intake and decreased thermogenesis.

as does stimulation of β_3-adrenoceptors with drugs such as Ro 16–8714[64]. Leptin synthesis and release are reduced in fasting, semi-starved and diabetic rats in parallel with reductions in white fat mass. Finally, endotoxin, tumour necrosis factor-α and interleukin-1 have recently been found to stimulate leptin production, suggesting a role for leptin in the anorexia seen in sepsis and cancer cachexia[65].

Other actions of leptin

Leptin has been demonstrated to inhibit insulin secretion by a direct action on pancreatic β-cells, which express leptin receptors[66], it has been suggested that leptin may form an 'adipoinsular' axis, which might limit lipogenesis by inhibition of insulin secretion[66]. Recently, leptin has been suggested to be involved with the development of insulin insensitivity that is seen in various obesity syndromes and diabetes (but clearly not the *ob/ob* mouse, which is markedly insulin resistant, yet lacks leptin). Leptin antagonises insulin action in the human hepatocellular carcinoma cell line HepG2, by interfering with early stages of receptor signalling; specifically it reduces insulin-induced tyrosine phosphorylation of IRS-1 (insulin receptor substrate-1) causing a reduction in binding of GRB-2 (growth factor-bound protein 2). In addition, leptin was able to antagonise insulin's ability to inhibit the synthesis of encoding phosphoenolpyruvate carboxykinase (PEPCK), the rate limiting enzyme in gluconeogenesis in a rat hepatoma cell line[67].

Leptin in human obesity

The discovery of leptin raised the possibility that human obesity, as in the *ob/ob* mouse, developed because of a failure to produce sufficient quantities of leptin. Indeed, an American biotechnology company have bought exclusive rights to develop leptin as an antiobesity treatment and clinical trials with leptin are underway. However, it is now clear that obese subjects, far from being leptin deficient, in fact have higher circulating levels of leptin than lean subjects, in proportion to their increased fat mass[68,69]. No equivalent abnormalities in the coding region of the human *OB* gene analogous to the *ob* mutation have been discovered in obese subjects, further suggesting that obesity does not develop from the inability to produce sufficient functional leptin. It is still possible that increasing the plasma concentration of leptin further in obese patients could reduce body weight. Evidence is emerging that leptin may be unable to reach its CNS sites of action in some obese humans; recent studies have demonstrated that the ratio of leptin concentrations in cerebrospinal fluid to plasma is disproportionally lower in obese subjects than in lean individuals[70]. This is perhaps because the transport system is already working at maximum capacity, or possibly because the leptin transport system has been attenuated in response to increased plasma leptin concentrations[63]. Although circulating leptin concentrations are increased in obese subjects they are not significantly different in diabetic subjects compared to controls. The suggestion, based on *in vitro* work, that the circulating leptin concentrations observed in obese and NIDDM subjects may contribute to the development of insulin sensitivity, needs to be confirmed by *in vivo* studies[67].

Regulation of food intake and body weight — the 'set point' hypothesis.

It has been proposed that each individual has a set point at which body weight and fat mass is regulated. However, it is clear both from a wealth of animal data and the rising prevalence of obesity in Westernised countries, that the set point is a range which is governed by various factors, and that it is possible to shift the set point by a number of mechanisms.

An individual's set point range is apparently determined by genetic factors, and (possibly) by factors such as intrauterine environment, resulting in programming of metabolism at birth[71]. The range within which an individual's body weight may change during life can be altered by major genetic defects such as leptin deficiency (e.g. the *ob/ob* mouse) or leptin resistance (e.g. the *db/db* mouse)[49,72]. Alternatively, there may be more minor polymorphisms in genes involved in body weight regulation such as the β_3-adrenoceptor gene and upstream mutations in the leptin gene which result in more subtle alterations in the set-point range[73–75].

Environmental factors are apparently able to shift the set point within an individual. For example, it is well recognised in rodents that exposure to highly palatable foods result in an increase in body weight[76]. This is akin to the concept of 'coca-colonization' in humans, when it is observed that rapid Westernization results in a massive increase in obesity in a population, as has been observed in Pacific islands such as Nauru. Other environmental factors include the level of physical activity, which may be a major determinant in the current epidemic of obesity which is being seen in the Western world (Fig. 5)[77].

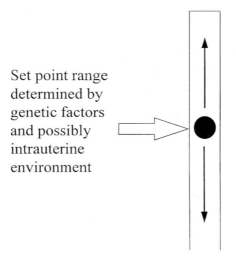

Fig. 5 Regulation of body weight—the 'set point' hypothesis. The set point is determined by genetic factors (such as β_3-adrenoceptor isoforms) and leptin. It can, however, be varied by alterations in diet, physical activity or with drugs.

Body weight regulation - the 'set point' model

Set point range determined by genetic factors and possibly intrauterine environment

- Sedentary lifestyle
- Food available
- High fat diet

- Physically active
- Low fat, high CHO diet
- Drugs?

Future strategies should include measures to alter correctable environmental factors such as physical activity and diet, and pharmacological agents which are able to shift the set point range within an individual. It is possible that agents modulating peripheral satiety signals such as CCK, central appetite-regulating mechanisms such as NPY, or long-term regulators of body weight such as leptin could all have a role.

References

1   Dryden S, Frankish H, Wang Q, Williams G. Neuropeptide Y and energy balance: one way ahead for the treatment of obesity? *Eur J Clin Invest* 1994; **24**: 293–308

2   Stanley BG, Kyrkouli SE, Lampert S, Leibowitz SF. Neuropeptide Y chronically injected into the hypothalamus: a powerful neurochemical inducer of hyperphagia and obesity. *Peptides* 1986; **7**: 1189–92

3   Stanley BG, Magdalin W, Seirafi A, Thomas WJ, Leibowitz SF. The perifornical area: the major focus of a patchily distributed hypothalamic neuropeptide Y sensitive feeding system(s). *Brain Res* 1993; **604**: 304–17

4   Wilding JPH. Metabolic actions of neuropeptide Y and their relevance to obesity. *Biochem Soc Trans* 1996; **24**: 576–81

5   Lambert PD, Wilding JPH, Al-Dokhayel AAM *et al*. A role for neuropeptide Y, dynorphin and noradrenaline in the central control of food intake after food deprivation. *Endocrinology* 1993; **133**: 29–32

6   McKibbin PE, Cotton SJ, McMillan S *et al*. Altered neuropeptide Y concentrations in specific hypothalmic regions of obese (*fa/fa*) Zucker rats—possible relationship to obesity and neuroendocrine disturbances. *Diabetes* 1991; **40**: 1423–9

7   Wilding JPH, Gilbey SG, Bailey CJ *et al*. Increased neuropeptide Y messenger RNA and decreased neurotensin messenger RNA in the hypothalamus of the obese (*ob/ob*) mouse. *Endocrinology* 1993; **132**: 1939–44

8   Dryden S, Pickavance L, Frankish HM, Williams G. Increased neuropeptide-Y secretion in the hypothalamic paraventricular nucleus of obese (*fa/fa*) Zucker rats. *Brain Res* 1995; **690**: 185–8

9   McCarthy HD, McKibbin PE, Holloway B, Mayers R, Williams G. Hypothalamic neuropeptide Y receptor characteristics and NPY-induced feeding responses in lean and obese Zucker rats. *Life Sci* 1991; **49**: 1491–7

10 Wilding JPH, Gilbey SG, Mannan M, Aslam N, Ghatei MA, Bloom SR. Increased neuropeptide Y content in individual hypothalamic nuclei, but not neuropeptide Y mRNA, in diet induced obesity in rats. *J Endocrinol* 1992; **132**: 299–304

11 Grundemar L, Hakanson R. Neuropeptide Y effector systems: perspectives for drug development. *Trends Pharmacol Sci* 1994; **15**: 153–9

12 Stanley BG, Magdalin W, Seirafi A, Nguyen MM, Leibowitz SF. Evidence for neuropeptide Y mediation of eating produced by food deprivation and for a variant of the Y1 receptor mediating this peptide's effect. *Peptides* 1992; **13**: 581–7

13 Gerald C, Walker MW, Criscione L *et al*. A receptor subtype involved in neuropeptide-Y-induced food-intake. *Nature* 1996; **382**: 168–171

14 Hu YH, Bloomquist BT, Cornfield LJ *et al*. Identification of a novel hypothalamic neuropeptide-Y receptor-associated with feeding-behavior. *J Biol Chem* 1996; **271**: 26315–9

15 Weinberg DH, Sirinathsinghji DJS, Tan CP *et al*. Cloning and expression of a novel neuropeptide-Y receptor. *J Biol Chem* 1996; **271**: 16435–8

16 Shor-Posner G, Grinker JA, Marinescu C, Brown O, Leibowitz SF. Hypothalamic serotonin in the control of meal patterns and macronutrient selection. *Brain Res Bull* 1986; **17**: 663–71

17 Kennett GA, Kurzon G. Evidence that hypophagia induced by mCPP and TFMPP requires 5-HT1c and 5-HT1d receptors; hypophagia induced by RU24969 only requires 5-HT1b receptors. *Psychopharmacology* 1988; **96**: 93–100

18 Bray GA, Ryan DH, Gordon D, Heidingsfelder S, Cerise F, Wilson K. Double-blind randomized placebo-controlled trial of sibutramine. *Obes Res* 1996; **4**: 263–70

19 Dryden S, Wang Q, Frankish HM, Pickavance L, Williams G. The serotonin (5-HT) antagonist methysergide increases neuropeptide-Y (NPY) synthesis and secretion in the hypothalamus of the rat. *Brain Res* 1995; **699**: 12–8

20 Dryden S, Wang QO, Frankish HM, Williams G. Differential-effects of the 5-HT1b/2c receptor agonist MCPP and the 5-HT1a agonist flesinoxan on hypothalamic neuropeptide-Y in the rat — evidence that NPY may mediate serotonins effects on food-intake. *Peptides* 1996; **17**: 943–9

21 Rogers P, McKibbin PE, Williams G. Acute fenfluramine administration reduces neuropeptide Y concentrations in specific hypothalmic regions of the rat: possible implications for the anorectic effect of fenfluramine. *Peptides* 1991; **12**: 251–5

22 Wilding JPH, Gilbey SG, Jones PM, Mannan MM, Ghatei MA, Bloom SR. Dexfenfluramine treatment and hypothalamic neuropeptides in diet-induced obesity in rats. *Peptides* 1992; **13**: 557–63

23 Mercer JG, Lawrence CB, Atkinson T. Hypothalamic *npy* and *crf* gene-expression in the food-deprived Syrian hamster. *Physiol Behav* 1996; **60**: 121–7

24 Appel NM, Owens MJ, Culp S *et al*. Role for brain corticotropin-releasing factor in the weight-reducing effects of chronic fenfluramine treatment in rats. *Endocrinology* 1991; **128**: 3237–46

25 Turton MD, O'Shea D, Gunn I *et al*. A role for glucagon-like peptide-1 in the central control of feeding. *Nature* 1996; **379**: 69–72

26 Gibbs J, Young RC, Smith GP. Cholecystokinin decreases food intake in rats. *J Comp Physiol Psychol* 1973; **84**: 488–95

27 Morley JE. Neuropeptide regulation of appetite and weight. *Endocr Rev* 1987; **8**: 256–87

28 Wank SA. Cholecystokinin receptors. *Am J Physiol* 1995; **32**: G628–G646

29 Dourish CT, Rycroft W, Iversen SD. Postponement of satiety by blockade of cholecystokinin (CCK-B) receptors. *Science* 1989; **245**: 1509–11

30 Ballinger AB, Mcloughlin L, Medbak S, Clark ML. Cholecystokinin is a satiety hormone at physiological post prandial concentrations. *Gastroenterology* 1994; **106**: A798

31 Lieverse RJ, Jansen JBMJ, Masclee AAM, Rovati LC, Lamers CBHW. Effect of a low-dose of intraduodenal fat on satiety in humans — studies using the type-a cholecystokinin receptor antagonist loxiglumide. *Gut* 1994; **35**: 501–5

32 Drewe J, Gadient A, Rovati LC, Beglinger C. Role of circulating cholecystokinin in control of fat-induced inhibition of food intake in humans. *Gastroenterology* 1992; **102**: 1654–9

33 Muurahainen NE, Kissileff HR, Pi-Sunyer FX. Intravenous infusion of bombesin reduces food intake in humans. *Am J Physiol* 1993; **264**: R350–R354

34 Gibbs J, Fauser DJ, Rowe EA, Rolls BJ, Rolls ET, Maddison SP. Bombesin suppresses feeding in rats. *Nature* 1979; **282**: 208–10

35 Stuckey JA, Gibbs J, Smith GP. Neural disconnection of gut from brain blocks bombesin induced satiety. *Peptides* 1985; **6**: 1249–52

36 Flynn FW. Fourth ventricular injection of selective bombesin receptor antagonists facilitates feeding in rats. *Am J Physiol* 1992; **264**: R218–R221

37 Porte D, Woods SC. Regulation of food intake and body weight by insulin. *Diabetologia* 1981; **20**: 274–80

38 McGowan MK, Andrews KM, Grossman SP. Chronic intrahypothalamic infusions of insulin or insulin antibodies alter body weight and food intake in the rat. *Physiol Behav* 1992; **51**: 753–66

39 Schwartz MW, Figlewicz DP, Baskin DG, Woods SC, Porte DJ. Insulin in the brain: a hormonal regulator of energy balance. *Endocr Rev* 1992; **13**: 387–414

40 Schwartz MW, Sipols AJ, Kahn SE *et al*. Kinetics and specificity of insulin uptake from plasma into cerebrospinal fluid. *Am J Physiol* 1990; **259**: E378–E383

41 Schwartz MW, Marks JL, Sipols AJ *et al*. Central insulin administration reduces neuropeptide-Y messenger RNA expression in the arcuate nucleus of food-deprived lean (FA/FA) but not obese (*fa/fa*) Zucker rats. *Endocrinology* 1991; **128**: 2645–7

42 Dubuc PU, Wilden NJ. Adrenalectomy reduces but does not reverse obesity in *ob/ob* mice. *Int J Obes* 1986; **10**: 91–8

43 Castonguay TW, Dallman MF, Stern JS. Some metabolic and behavioural effects of adrenalectomy on obese Zucker rats. *Am J Physiol* 1986; **251**: R923–R933

44 Debons AF, Zurek LD, Tse CS, Abrahamsen S. Central nervous system control of hyperphagia in hypothalamic obesity: dependence on adrenal glucocorticoids. *Endocrinology* 1986; **118**: 1678–81

45 Stanley BG, Lanthier D, Chin AS, Leibowitz SF. Suppression of neuropeptide Y-elicited eating by adrenalectomy or hypophysectomy: reversal with corticosterone. *Brain Res* 1989; **501**: 32–6

46 Wilding JPH, Gilbey SG, Lambert PD, Ghatei MA, Bloom SR. Increases in neuropeptide Y content and gene expression in the hypothalamus of rats treated with dexamethasone are prevented by insulin. *Neuroendocrinology* 1993; **57**: 581–7

47 Kennedy GC. The role of depot fat in the hypothalamic regulation of food intake in the rat. *Proc R Soc Lond [Biol]* 1953; **140**: 578–92

48 Coleman DL. Effects of parabiosis of obese with diabetes and normal mice. *Diabetologia* 1973; **9**: 294–8

49 Zhang YY, Proenca R, Maffei M, Barone M, Leopold L, Friedman JM. Positional cloning of the mouse obese gene and its human homolog. *Nature* 1994; **372**: 425–32

50 Levin N, Nelson C, Gurney A, Vandlen R, DeSauvage F. Decreased food intake does not completely account for adiposity reduction after ob protein infusion. *Proc Natl Acad Sci USA* 1996; **93**: 1726–30

51 Halaas JL, Gajiwala KS, Maffei M et al. Weight-reducing effects of the plasma protein encoded by the obese gene. *Science* 1995; **269**: 543–6

52 Mercer JG, Hoggard N, Williams LM et al. Coexpression of leptin receptor and preproneuropeptide-Y messenger-RNA in arcuate nucleus of mouse hypothalamus. *J Neuroendocrinol* 1996; **8**: 733–5

53 Banks WA, Kastin AJ, Huang WT, Jaspan JB, Maness LM. Leptin enters the brain by a saturable system independent of insulin. *Peptides* 1996; **17**: 305–11

54 Malik KF, Young WS. Localization of binding-sites in the central-nervous-system for leptin (ob protein) in normal, obese (*ob/ob*), and diabetic (*db/db*) c57bl/6j mice. *Endocrinology* 1996; **137**: 1497–500

55 Tartaglia LA, Dembski M, Weng X et al. Identification and expression cloning of a leptin receptor, ob-r. *Cell* 1995; **83**: 1263–71

56 Lee GH, Proenca R, Montez JM et al. Abnormal splicing of the leptin receptor in diabetic mice. *Nature* **1996**; **379**: 632–5

57 Chen H, Charlat O, Tartaglia LA et al. Evidence that the diabetes gene encodes the leptin receptor — identification of a mutation in the leptin receptor gene in *db/db* mice. *Cell* 1996; **84**: 491–5

58 Phillips MS, Liu QY, Hammond HA et al. Leptin receptor missense mutation in the fatty zucker rat. *Nature Genet* 1996; **13**: 18–9

59 Baumann H, Morella KK, White DW et al. The full-length leptin receptor has signaling capabilities of interleukin 6-type cytokine receptors. *Proc Natl Acad Sci USA* 1996; **93**: 8374–8

60 Stephens TW, Basinski M, Bristow PK et al. The role of neuropeptide Y in the antiobesity action of the obese gene product. *Nature* 1995; **377**: 530–2

61 Wang Q, Bing C, Al-Barazanji K et al. Interactions between leptin and hypothalamic neuropeptide Y neurons in the control of food intake and energy homeostasis in the rat. *Diabetes* 1997; In press

62 Erickson JC, Hollopeter G, Palmiter RD. Attenuation of the obesity syndrome of *ob/ob* mice by the loss of neuropeptide-Y. *Science* 1996; **274**: 1704–7

63 Frederich RC, Hamann A, Anderson S, Lollmann B, Lowell BB, Flier JS. Leptin levels reflect body lipid-content in mice — evidence for diet-induced resistance to leptin action. *Nature Med* 1995; **1**: 1311–4

64 Slieker LJ, Sloop KW, Surface PL et al. Regulation of expression of ob messenger-RNA and protein by glucocorticoids and cAMP. *J Biol Chem* 1996; **271**: 5301–4

65 Grunfeld C, Zhao C, Fuller J et al. Endotoxin and cytokines induce expression of leptin, the *ob* gene-product, in hamsters — a role for leptin in the anorexia of infection. *J Clin Invest* 1996; **97**: 2152–7

66 Kieffer TJ, Heller RS, Habener JF. Leptin receptors expressed on pancreatic beta-cells. *Biochem Biophys Res Commun* 1996; **224**: 522–7

67 Cohen B, Novick D, Rubinstein M. Modulation of insulin activities by leptin. *Science* 1996; **274**: 1185–8

68 Klein S, Coppack SW, Mohamed-Ali V, Landt M. Adipose tissue leptin production and plasma leptin kinetics in humans. *Diabetes* 1996; **45**: 984–6

69 Considine RV, Sinha MK, Heiman ML *et al*. Serum immunoreactive leptin concentrations in normal-weight and obese humans. *N Engl J Med* 1996; **334**: 292–5

70 Schwartz MW, Peskind E, Raskind M, Boyko EJ, Porte D. Cerebrospinal-fluid leptin levels — relationship to plasma-levels and to adiposity in humans. *Nature Med* 1996; **2**: 589–93

71 Hales CN, Barker DJP. Type 2 (non-insulin dependent) diabetes mellitus: the thrifty phenotype hypothesis. *Diabetologia* 1992; **35**: 595–601

72 Chua SC, Chung WK, Wupeng XS *et al*. Phenotypes of mouse diabetes and rat fatty due to mutations in the ob (leptin) receptor. *Science* 1996; **271**: 994–6

73 Reed DR, Ding Y, Xu WZ, Cather C, Green ED, Price RA. Extreme obesity may be linked to markers flanking the human *ob* gene. *Diabetes* 1996; **45**: 691–4

74 Clement K, Garner C, Hager J *et al*. Indication for linkage of the human *ob* gene region with extreme obesity. *Diabetes* 1996; **45**: 687–90

75 Arner P. The beta(3)-adrenergic receptor — a cause and cure of obesity. *N Engl J Med* 1995; **333**: 382–3

76 Sclafani A, Springer D. Dietary obesity in adult rats: similarities to hypothalamic and human obesity syndromes. *Physiol Behav* 1976; **17**: 461–71

77 Prentice AM, Jebb SA. Obesity in britain — gluttony or sloth. *BMJ* 1995; **311**: 437–9

Obesity as a disease

Roland T Jung

The Diabetic Centre, Ninewells Hospital, Dundee, UK

Obesity is associated with the development of some of the most prevalent diseases of modern society. The greatest risk is for diabetes mellitus where a body mass index above 35 kg/m² increases the risk by 93-fold in women and by 42-fold in men. The risk of coronary heart disease is increased 86% by a 20% rise in weight in males, whereas in obese women the risk is increased 3.6-fold. Elevation of blood pressure, hyperlipidaemia and altered haemostatic factors are implicated in this high risk from coronary heart disease. Gallbladder disease is increased 2.7-fold with an enhanced cancer risk especially for colorectal cancer in males and cancer of the endometrium and biliary passages in females. Endocrine changes are associated with metabolic diseases and infertility, and respiratory problems result in sleep apnoea, hypoventilation, arrhythmias and eventual cardiac failure. Obesity is not a social stigma but an actual disease with a major genetic component to its aetiology and a financial cost estimated at $69 billion for the USA alone.

Obesity is not just a health risk but a disease. Estimates of the genetic contribution to weight gain in susceptible families range from 25–40% with a greater heritability for abdominal fat distribution of 50%[1,2]. Obviously there is a major environmental effect but this genetic susceptibility alone removes this condition from a social stigma to the disease category. The many associated conditions, such as diabetes, which are directly attributable to excessive weight make obesity a major influence on disease progression and, with its high prevalence, places obesity as the major nutritional disease of the Westernised world. This chapter describes those diseases associated with obesity by reference to mortality and morbidity and also by emphasising the advantage to health and co-morbid risk factors of weight loss.

Mortality

Correspondence to:
Dr Roland T Jung,
Diabetic Centre,
Ninewells Hospital and
Medical School,
Dundee DD1 9SY, UK

There is now extensive evidence that links excessive body weight with overall mortality. The overall relationship between mortality and body mass index (BMI) adjusted for age shows a J shaped curve (Fig. 1) with an acceleration of the mortality risk above a BMI of 30[3]. This is well illustrated by the work of Manson *et al*.[4] who examined the association between BMI and both overall mortality and mortality from specific diseases in a cohort of 115,195 women from the USA enrolled in their prospective Nurses' Health Study. These women were 30–55 years of age and healthy when enrolled in 1976. During 16 years of follow-up, there were 4726 deaths, some 881 from cardiovascular causes, 2586 from cancer and 1259 from other aetiologies. In the analysis of those women who had never smoked, the increased relative risk of death is not only seen in those with frank obesity but the risk rises with modest gains in weight. For instance, the increased relative risk of death was 1.3 in those with a BMI 25.0–26.9, 1.6 in those with a BMI 27.0–28.9 and was doubled (2.1) for those with a BMI of 29.0–31.9. Among women with a BMI above 32 who had never smoked, the risk of death from cardiovascular disease was 4.1 and from cancer was 2.1. In terms of attributable risk, some 53% of all deaths in this study among women with a BMI of 29 or greater could be attributed directly to their obesity.

Some have described the relationship between mortality and BMI as a J shaped curve with a rising mortality in the thinnest individuals[3]. This apparent excess risk associated with leanness was found to be artifactual in the above nurses' study and was eliminated after accounting for smoking and subclinical disease[4]. With these exclusions, lean women (BMI < 19) had the lowest mortality. However, a weight gain of 10 kg or more from the age of 18 years was associated with an increased mortality in middle age. In contrast, those women who lost weight or gained less than 10 kg did not have a significant change in mortality. Also the BMI at age 18 years predicted overall and cardiovascular mortality in middle age[4].

Although coronary heart disease is a major cause of weight-related death, the obese often develop other conditions which further predispose to their mortality. This relative mortality is highest for diabetes mellitus and next for digestive diseases including cancer. Table 1 shows this relative mortality risk of obesity reported in a study of 750,000 men and women by Lew and Garfinkel[5]. In this study, the mortality for cancer was highest for colorectal cancer in males (1.73 in males, 1.22 in females), whereas in females this was in endometrial cancer followed by cancer of the gallbladder and biliary passages. In addition, those with substantial obesity had an increased risk of cervix, breast and ovarian cancers.

Smoking appreciably elevates mortality (Fig. 1) such that those who smoke 20 or more cigarettes per day have double the risk of non-smokers throughout the weight range and this is especially apparent in males. Cessation of smoking often results in weight gain; in one study this averaged 2.8 kg in males and 3.8 kg in females[6]. Weight gain results from a decrease in energy expenditure (each cigarette utilises 8 kcal by stimulation of the sympathetic system) and also by enhanced energy

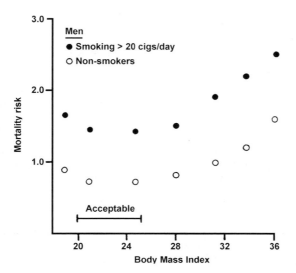

Fig. 1 Mortality risk across a range of body mass indices in males[3]. The risk of smoking 20 cigarettes per day is shown. The mortality risk of a smoker of acceptable weight is similar to an obese man of BMI 35 kg/m² who does not smoke. On smoking cessation, a weight gain of 11–13 kg would be required to negate the mortality advantage of the non-smoker.

intake. The priority should always be to advise cessation of smoking for the health risk is greater. A weight gain of as much as 11–13 kg would be required to equate to the same mortality risk as a non-smoker. In one study this amount of weight was gained by 9.8% of males and 13.4% of females on cessation of smoking indicating that, although the majority will benefit, there is also a need for parallel dietary advice[6].

Recent evidence indicates that a weight loss of more than 9 kg in women is associated with a 25% reduction in all causes (diabetic, cardiovascular and cancer) of mortality[7]. If the obese person has already developed a weight related disease, then intentional weight loss of any amount has been shown to reduce mortality by 20%. This is most marked for cancer (with a 40–50% reduction) and for diabetes (with a

Table 1 Mortality risk in obesity. Compares the risk of those weighing 140% or more above an ideal weight (100%) with those weighing 90–109% of ideal[5]

	Males	Females
Diabetes mellitus	5.19	7.90
Digestive diseases	3.99	2.29
Coronary heart disease	1.85	2.07
Cerebral vascular disease	2.27	1.52
Cancer: all sites	1.33	1.55
Cancer: colorectal	1.73	
Cancer: prostate	1.29	
Cancer: gallbladder/biliary		3.58
Cancer: endometrium		5.42
Cancer: cervix		2.39
Cancer: ovary		1.63

Table 2 Morbidity in obesity

Cardiovascular	Hypertension	**Breast**	Breast cancer
	Coronary heart disease		Male gynaecomastia
	Cerebrovascular disease	**Uterus**	Endometrial cancer
	Varicose veins		Cervical cancer
	Deep venous thrombosis	**Urological**	Prostate cancer
	Hypertension		Stress incontinence
Respiratory	Breathless	**Skin**	Sweat rashes
	Sleep apnoea		Fungal infections
	Hypoventilation syndrome		Lymphoedema
Gastrointestinal	Hiatus hernia		Cellulitis
	Gallstones and cholelithiasis		Acanthosis nigracans
	Fatty liver and cirrhosis	**Orthopaedic**	Osteoarthritis
	Haemorrhoids		Gout
	Herniae	**Endocrine**	Growth hormone and IGF1 reduced
	Cancer colorectal		Reduced prolactin response
Metabolic	Hyperlipidaemia		Hyperdynamic ACTH response to CRH
	Insulin resistance		Increased urinary free cortisol
	Diabetes mellitus		Altered sex hormones
	Polycystic ovarian syndrome	**Pregnancy**	Obstetric complications
	Hyperandrogenisation		Caesarean operation
	Menstrual irregularities		Large babies
Neurology	Nerve entrapment		Neural tube defects
Renal	Proteinuria		

30–40% fall in mortality). It is important to emphasise 'intentional' weight loss, for much confusion has arisen in the past from the inclusion of non-intentional, i.e. disease driven, weight loss which pre-empts death from many conditions.

Morbidity

Excess weight is associated with a multiplicity of problems[8] as outlined in Table 2, hence the categorisation in many countries of obesity as a distinct disease. Equally, a 10 kg weight loss can confer significant health benefits (Table 3).

Diabetes mellitus

Most non insulin dependent diabetic patients are overweight, about 75% in most studies. Colditz *et al.*[9] have reported on the development of diabetes in females in a 14 year prospective study of 114,281 nurses aged 30–55 years who did not have this condition or coronary heart disease, stroke or cancer at the outset. After adjustment for age, BMI was the dominant predictor of the risk for diabetes. In females the risk rises

Table 3   Benefits of a 10 kg weight loss

Mortality	20–25% fall in total mortality
	30–40% fall in diabetes related deaths
	40–50% fall in obesity related cancer deaths
Blood pressure	Fall of 10 mmHg systolic pressure
	Fall of 20 mmHg diastolic pressure
Angina	Reduced symptoms by 91%
	33% increase in exercise tolerance
Lipids	Fall by 10% in total cholesterol
	Fall by 15% in LDL cholesterol
	Fall by 30% in triglycerides
	Increase by 8% in HDL cholesterol
Diabetes	Reduces risk of developing diabetes by > 50%
	Fall of 30–50% in fasting blood glucose
	Fall of 15% in HbA1c

above a BMI of 22 with a 5-fold increased risk at a BMI of 25, 28-fold risk at BMI of 30 and a 93-fold higher risk above a BMI of 35. Compared to those of stable weight, a gain of 8–10.9 kg increases the risk of diabetes by 2.7-fold. In contrast, those women who lose more than 5 kg, reduce their risk of developing diabetes by 50% or more. These results were also independent of any family history of diabetes.

The situation in males was reported by Chan *et al.*[10] in a study of 51,529 men aged 40–75 years in 1986 and subsequently followed up for 5 years. Increased risk was seen for all BMI levels of 24 or above. Even men with a slight excess weight were more likely to develop diabetes than those with a BMI less than 23 kg/m^2. The risk adjusted for age was increased 2.2-fold in those with BMI 25–26.9, 6.7 in those with BMI 29–30.9 and 42 in those with BMI of 35 or more. The BMI at age 21 years and the absolute weight gain during adulthood were independent risk factors for diabetes development. A BMI of 27 at age 21 years increased the risk 6.4-fold whereas a gain in weight of 9 kg from the age of 21 years further raised the risk 3.5-fold. Fat distribution measured by the waist circumference was also independently associated with diabetes development. A waist above 40 inches (100 cm) alone increased the risk by 3.5-fold even after control for BMI.

These results are in keeping with a major study in Oslo by Westlund and Nicolayson[11] on the 10 year follow up of 3751 men aged 40–49 years at the outset. The percentage developing diabetes was 0.6% in normal weight men but 23.4% in those 25% or more overweight. Weight loss improves this risk in males and females. In the nurses' study reported above, a 5 kg weight loss reduced the risk of developing diabetes by 50% or more. Weight loss also improves mortality in those with established diabetes. A 9 kg weight loss reduces diabetes related mortality by 30–40%[7], whereas a 5% weight loss reduces HbA1C by 7% and decreases fasting blood glucose by 15%[12]. A loss of 10–20% in weight in non insulin dependent diabetic patients can normalise metabolic control and possibly life expectancy.

Cardiovascular disease, blood pressure, lipids and rheology

A number of cardiovascular risk factors are influenced by overweight including hypertension, impaired glycaemic control, dyslipidaemia and haemostatic and rheological factors. Until recently it was thought that only severe degrees of excess weight increased the risk of *coronary heart disease* but recent evidence shows a clear association with modest weight gain. In the nurses' study, Willett *et al.*[13] controlled for age, smoking, menopausal status, post menopausal hormone use and family history. They found that the risk of coronary heart disease was increased 2-fold in those women of BMI 25–28.9 and 3.6 for a BMI of 29 or more. Weight gain from age 18 years increased the risk 1.6-fold for a 8–10.9 kg gain and 1.9-fold for a 11–19 kg gain. In males, a 10% increase in weight will increase the risk of coronary heart disease by 38% whereas a 20% weight rise corresponds with a 86% increased risk[3].

Blood pressure is increased by 6 mm systolic and 4 mm diastolic for a 10% gain in body fat with those genetically more susceptible showing the greater effect. Reisen *et al.*[14] have demonstrated that a weight loss of 11 kg produced a 20% decrease in both systolic and diastolic pressure in hypertensive patients even when the sodium intake was kept constant. It would appear that, as a general rule, blood pressure is reduced by 1 mm systolic and 2 mm diastolic for each 1% reduction in body weight.

The most characteristic *lipid disorder* in obesity is elevated total cholesterol and triglycerides, high LDL-cholesterol and low HDL-cholesterol. A meta-analysis by Datillo and Kris-Etherton[15] of some 70 published studies and other work reviewed, has indicated that for every 1 kg of weight lost, there is a corresponding reduction by about 1% in total cholesterol and LDL, a rise by 1% in HDL and a reduction by 3% of triglycerides.

A number of *haemostatic factors* are associated with weight gain, particularly factors VII and X which may relate to thrombosis and the risk of fatal myocardial infarction. In a study by Ernst and Matrai[16] using a 4.2 MJ diet, a 15% weight loss was associated with a decrease by 27% in blood viscosity, by 20% in red cell aggregation and by 5.5% in haematocrit; plasma fibrinogen remained unaffected. Hankey *et al.*[17] have shown that a 5 kg weight loss reduced both factor VII coagulant activity and red cell aggregability by 10%, whereas a weight loss of 5% can improve plasma activator inhibitor by 42%[18].

Such data on blood pressure, lipids and haemostatic factors most likely account for the reduction in morbidity and mortality from cardiovascular diseases with modest weight loss. In one study by Ornish et al.[19] a 10 kg weight loss over 1 year reduced symptoms of angina by 91% with a 33% increase in exercise tolerance. The St Thomas Atherosclerosis Regression Study has shown the benefit of a reduced fat intake with or without cholestyramine on atheroma progression[20]. The luminal diameter widened in 38% on a reduced fat intake diet, in 33% in those on diet and cholestyramine but in only 4% in the control group. The corresponding figures for coronary heart disease progression were 15% on reduced fat diet, 12% on diet and cholestyramine but 46% in the controls. An important feature of this trial was that weight loss was part of therapy in those with a BMI above 25. Ornish et al.[19] also reported a 8.8% reduction in atheroma on polyvalent therapy including weight loss. These studies suggest that weight loss might reduce atheroma and may account for the 9% reduction in cardiovascular disease mortality reported with weight loss in the study of 43,457 women by Williamson et al.[7].

Obesity causes left ventricular hypertrophy which can co-exist with the cardiac changes associated with essential hypertension[21]. In early stages of hypertension, cardiac output and peripheral resistance are both elevated, increasing blood pressure. Further increases in peripheral resistance caused by excess smooth muscle contraction and a contracted intravascular volume result in a progressive blood pressure rise with the result that the heart compensates for the increased afterload by left ventricular myocyte thickening and lengthening in a **concentric** manner. In obesity, the increased lean mass, fat mass, body surface area and metabolic rate are associated with increased oxygen consumption resulting in an increased cardiac output by a rise in stroke volume. As total blood and plasma volume are also expanded, there is an increase in preload with an increased left ventricular end-diastolic volume resulting in left ventricular chamber dilatation. Cardiovascular reserve is preserved by compensatory hypertrophy of the left ventricle in an **eccentric** manner so that the ratio between wall thickness and the chamber cavity radius is preserved (unlike hypertension where it is increased). If the obese become hypertensive then the resultant increased afterload can result in cardiac dilatation and hypertrophy and clinical cardiac failure. Left ventricular hypertrophy can be anticipated in more than 50% of patients who are more than 50% overweight[22].

Cerebrovascular disease is common in the obese. In the Whitehall study involving 17,753 men aged 40–64 years, the risk associated with obesity for death from a stroke was more apparent in younger subjects and nonsmokers[23]. In men aged 40–54 years, the most obese quintile had a mortality ratio some 2-fold higher than the thinnest. However, in men aged 55–64 years this ratio was only 1.2. The increased risk was more apparent in nonsmokers where the age adjusted ratio was 2.6. The Chicago stroke study of a biracial cohort aged 65–74 years did not show an association between body weight alone and stroke when potential confounders were controlled for in the analysis such as black race, female gender, age 70+, hypertension and diabetes all of which were independently associated with risk of stroke[24]. Shinton et al.[25] have compared 125 men and women who had a first stroke and aged 35–74 years with 198 age and sex matched controls. They found an association between highest quartile for BMI and stroke with an odds ratio after multiple risk factor adjustment of 2.25. This lifelong pattern of risk appeared to be established early for the risk factor adjusted odds ratio for the BMI at age 21 years was 2.13.

Digestive diseases

Gallbladder disease is the most common form of digestive disease in obese individuals. Rimm et al.[26], in a study of 73,532 obese women in USA and Canada, reported a 2.7-fold increase in the prevalence of gallbladder disease. There is a progressive linear increased risk of gallstones from a BMI of 20 upwards which is twice as high in women as in men which further increases with age, and the number of pregnancies[27]. Weight and age appear additive with obesity being 6-fold more important than age[28]. Weight loss may actually exacerbate gallbladder disease. In the Boston nurses' study, women who lost 4–10 kg had a 44% increased risk for detectable gallstone disease, whereas weight loss above 10 kg increased this risk to 94%[29]. The reason for this may be associated with the rise in the body pool of circulating cholesterol as adipose tissue stores are mobilised and the increase in rate at which cholesterol is excreted in the bile as obesity develops. The development of gallstones depends on the precipitation of cholesterol from a supersaturated bile. Dieting using inadequate dietary fibre further decreases the solubilisation of excreted cholesterol increasing gallstone formation.

Liver abnormalities have been described in the obese mainly due to fatty infiltration. However, in the morbidly obese with BMI greater than 40, one study[30] found only 2% had normal livers, 56% showed fatty infiltration alone, whereas 42% had fatty infiltration associated with fibrosis or cirrhosis. In the American Cancer Society study[5] of 750,000 men and women in the USA followed for 12 years, colorectal cancer was the principal site of excess cancer mortality in obese males (relative rates: 1.73 in males, 1.22 in females), whereas in obese females the highest prevalence was from cancer of the gallbladder and biliary passages (relative mortality of 3.6). The relative mortality rates of cancer of the stomach and pancreas were higher in obese males (1.88 and 1.62, respectively) than in females where the mortality rate for stomach cancer (1.03) was reported similar to the non-obese and that for pancreatic cancer (0.61) significantly lower. The relative risk of endometrial cancer is more than doubled in women aged 60–69 years with a BMI of 25–29 kg/m^2 and is increased 5.4-fold in those with significant obesity[5,31].

Breast cancer

The relationship between breast cancer and obesity is not clear[32]. In the American Cancer Society study, the mortality ratio for breast cancer was not significantly raised for those 120–139% above ideal body weight (IBW = 100%), but was 1.63 for those greater than 140% IBW[5]. However, age has a significant impact on the risk of developing breast cancer. Premenopausal obese women have the same risk as lean women but in the postmenopause, obese women exhibit a higher risk[33]. Abdominal obesity and a positive family history increase this risk. It has been conjectured that this association with obesity, and especially central adiposity, is associated with enhanced conversion of androgens to oestrogen in the fat mass and a reduced sex-hormone binding globulin (SHBG) which adds to an increase in free oestradiol levels.

Lung cancer

This is one cancer which the obese are less prone to develop. The adjusted odds ratio for non smokers with BMI <22 was 2.9 in women and 0.9 in males compared to those with BMI <28. The odds ratio for smokers in the group with BMI <22 was 2.0 in both sexes[34].

Arthritis and bone mass

It is not easy to find objective evidence for the improvement of arthritis with weight loss especially in the elderly. Whereas there is evidence that obesity is associated with osteoarthritis of the hip and knee, extensive literature does not indicate that weight loss in modest obesity had any measurable clinical benefit on this condition. In contrast McGoey et al.[35]

have reported that in the morbidly obese there is relief of pain in the lower back, ankles and feet with 6–10 kg weight loss. Bone mass is increased in the obese but bone mass can decrease by 3–15% with weight loss[36]. Some suggest that this loss recovers with weight regain, but not necessarily in postmenopausal women. Uric acid levels also increase with weight, precipitating gout, and also acutely rise with dieting. Musculoskeletal problems result in increased disability and the need for time off work, seen even in those with modest overweight[37].

Endocrine abnormalities and psychological factors

The production of sex steroids is altered in the obese[38]. Obese women, especially those with central adiposity, have increased levels of free testosterone and are hyperandrogenic with marked insulin resistance, the latter implicated in the development of polycystic ovarian syndrome. In obese men, visceral adiposity is associated with a reduced testosterone level. Growth hormone is also reduced in obesity and insulin-like growth factor (IGF-1) is negatively associated with increasing visceral adiposity[39]. Some obese women also show a reduced prolactin stimulatory response associated with a reduced catecholamine rise to insulin induced hypoglycaemia[40]. It has been conjectured that these hormonal abnormalities may be secondary to an increased activity of the hypothalamic-pituitary axis. Corticotrophin-releasing hormone (CRH) which stimulates the secretion of ACTH from the pituitary has also been reported to inhibit both growth hormone releasing hormone and gonadotrophin releasing hormone which influence IGF-1 and sex steroids respectively as well as inducing insulin resistance[38].

Those who have visceral obesity exhibit a hyperdynamic ACTH secretion to CRH, as well as increased cortisol release from the adrenals, whereas those with gynaecoid obesity show a lesser response, identical to that observed in naturally thin individuals[41]. Urinary free cortisol levels have also been reported to be positively associated with increasing visceral adiposity[42]. As cortisol and insulin both increase fat accumulation, whereas growth hormone and testosterone promote lipid metabolism, the abnormalities noted in the obese would have the effect of promoting fat deposition, especially of visceral fat.

This overactivity of the hypothalamic pituitary axis has been conjectured as due to higher, cortical, influences possibly related to certain socioeconomic factors and psychological problems which appear to be more prevalent in the visceral obese. In population studies, men and women with a higher waist–hip ratio (more visceral obesity) report ill more often, have more frequent peptic ulcers and stomach bleeding and have more general health complaints[38]. These individuals use more tranquillisers and antidepressant tablets, have more time off work for sickness, suffer stress related symptoms, sleeplessness and nightmares. They tend to be from the lower socio-economic groups, have poorer education, impaired personality, extra-version, low achievement, aggression, low dominance and have a need for sociability. Such inability to cope with life events in those with a genetic propensity for a certain fat distribution may produce a permanent hyperarousal response which stimulates certain brain peptides, especially CRH, which then drive the pituitary adrenal axis to produce a raised cortisol output[43]. Such would also be implicated in neuropeptide Y release, one of the brain's most potent peptides for the stimulation of appetite especially for carbohydrates. This peptide could potentiate CRH release producing a vicious cycle driving the individual onwards to store visceral fat[38].

Studies into the effects of stress on hormonal levels in monkeys replicate the above scenario[44]. If the social hierarchy of the monkey colony is deliberately disrupted to induce a helplessness reaction to stress, then the monkeys accumulate visceral fat with increased cortisol secretion, large adrenals, low sex steroid levels, insulin resistance and coronary heart disease.

Respiratory problems

There are a number of ways in which obesity affects lung function[45]. An increased amount of fat in the chest wall and abdomen limits respiratory excursion reducing lung volume. This is accentuated in the supine position increasing the mechanical work of breathing by 30% in modest obesity and by a 3-fold increase in obesity-hypoventilation syndrome (sometimes called the Pickwickian syndrome). A ventilation/perfusion disturbance resulting in abnormal gas exchange is often observed in extremes of obesity, with underventilated but overperfused lower portions of the lungs. This results in hypoxia with normal arterial carbon dioxide levels, the degree of hypoxia worsening in the supine position. This hypoxia expands the pulmonary blood volume which adds strain to ventricular function. These changes in respiratory function are most important during sleep. During rapid eye movement (REM) sleep, there are decreases in voluntary muscle tone with a reduction in arterial oxygen saturation and a rise in carbon dioxide tension in all individuals, but especially marked in the obese. Irregular respiration and occasional apnoeic episodes often occur in lean people during REM sleep, but obesity with its influence on respiratory mechanics increases their frequency and may result in severe hypoxia with resultant arrhythmias and cardiac dysfunction.

In many with uncomplicated obesity, these ventilation perfusion defects are countered by increased ventilation which restores blood gases to normal, but in some there develops depression in both hypercapnic and hypoxic respiratory drives and with an accompanying irregular pattern of breathing with apnoeic episodes can result in obesity-hypoventilation syndrome. As their obesity worsens, so do the apnoeic episodes resulting in frequent awakening and the resultant sleep deprivation produces daytime somnolence[45]. Persistent hypoxia further blunts the hypoxic drive resulting in a deteriorating cycle with the development of pulmonary hypertension and eventual right ventricular failure worsening the hypoxia. 24 h monitoring of arterial oxygen saturation using an ear lobe oximeter will help in the diagnosis of those at risk.

Pregnancy

Obese women have a higher risk of obstetric complications. The relative risk of antenatal complications in women whose prepregnancy weight was at least 135% of IBW was reported increased 6.6-fold for the development of diabetes, 1.9-fold for pregnancy induced hypertension and 1.4-fold for urinary tract infections[46]. Other complications include pre-eclampsia (1.5-fold risk), thrombophlebitis, post partum haemorrhage and wound or episiotomy infections. Obese women have an increased risk of Caesarean delivery due to a variety of factors, such as fetal size especially macrosomia (birth weights >4000 g), an increase in maternal pelvic soft tissue narrowing the birth canal, late deceleration of the fetal heart rate, intrapartum meconium staining, prolonged labour, malpresentations and cord incidents[47]. This increased prevalence of Caesarean section occurs in pregnancies with or without antenatal complications. In the latter, the rate has been reported as high as 19.6% in the morbidly obese compared to 10.1% in normal weight and 12.4% in moderate obesity[47]. Fetal weight appears to be directly proportional to maternal size with more than 50% of obese women having babies who weigh greater than 3600 g. Maternal weight when not associated with antenatal complications is not associated with an increased perinatal mortality, but this is increased if there is an antenatal complication by as much as 3-fold[47,48]. Recently, an increased risk of neural tube defects, especially spina bifida, has been reported in women with BMI greater than 29 (odds ratio 1.9)[49].

Conclusion

Obesity is a disease associated with extensive human suffering and also a massive financial cost to society. It has been estimated that for the year 1990, the direct cost of obesity associated disease in the USA alone was $45.8 billion and the indirect costs $23 billion[50]. Hence the total economic cost of obesity in USA was estimated as $68.8 billion[50]. At such a cost to society, obesity is not a social condition but a rampant disease. Obesity is not simply a matter of overeating and lack of will power but a disease with a major genetic aetiology modified by the environment and should be treated vigorously in the same manner that we now apply to its associated co-morbid conditions such as diabetes, coronary heart disease, hypertension and hyperlipidaemia.

References

1   Bouchard C, Perusse L. Genetics of obesity. *Annu Rev Nutr* 1993; **13**: 337–54
2   Sorensen TIA. The genetics of obesity. *Metabolism* 1995; **44 Suppl 3**: 4–6
3   Royal College of Physicians. Obesity. *J R Coll Physicians Lond* 1983; **17**: 3–58
4   Manson JE, Willett WC, Stampfer MJ *et al*. Body weight and mortality among women. *N Engl J Med* 1995; **333**: 677–85
5   Lew EA, Garfinkel L. Variations in mortality by weight among 750,000 men and women. *J Chronic Dis* 1979; **32**: 563–76
6   Williamson DF, Madans J, Anda RF, Kleinman JC, Giovino GA, Byers T. Smoking cessation and severity of weight gain in a national cohort. *N Engl J Med* 1991; **324**: 739–45
7   Williamson DF, Pamuk E, Thun M, Flanders D, Byers T, Heath C. Prospective study of intentional weight loss and mortality in never smoking overweight US white women aged 40–64 years. *Am J Epidemiol* 1995; **141**: 1128–41
8   Jung RT. *A Colour Atlas of Obesity*. London: Wolfe Medical Publications, 1990
9   Colditz GA, Willett WC, Rotnitzky A, Manson JE. Weight gain as a risk factor for clinical diabetes mellitus in women. *Ann Intern Med* 1995; **122**: 481–6
10 Chan JM, Stampfer MJ, Rimm EB, Willett WC, Colditz GA. Obesity, fat distribution, and weight gain as risk factors for clinical diabetes in men. *Diabetes Care* 1994; **17**: 961–9
11 Westlund K, Nicolayson R. A ten year mortality and morbidity study related to serum cholesterol. A follow-up of 3751 men aged 40–49. *Scand J Lab Invest* 1972; **30 Suppl 127**: 1–24
12 Wing RR, Shoemaker M, Marcus MDM, McDermott M, Gooding W. Variables associated with weight loss and improvements in glycaemic control in type 2 diabetic patients. *Arch Intern Med* 1990; **147**: 1749–53
13 Willett WC, Manson JE, Stampfer MJ *et al*. Weight, weight change and coronary heart disease in women. *JAMA* 1995; **27**: 1461–5
14 Reisen E, Abel R, Modan M, Silverberg DS, Eliahou HE, Modan B. The effect of weight loss without salt restriction on the reduction in blood pressure in overweight hypertensive patients. *N Engl J Med* 1978; **298**: 1–6
15 Dattilo AM, Kris-Etherton PM. Effects of weight reduction on blood lipids and lipoproteins: a meta analysis. *Am J Clin Nutr* 1992; **56**: 320–8
16 Ernst E, Matrai A. Normalisation of hemorreological abnormalities during weight reduction in obese patients. *Nutrition* 1987; **3**: 337–9
17 Hankey CR, Rumley A, Lowe GDO, Lean MEJ. Weight loss improves established indices of ischaemic heart disease risk. *Proc Nutr Soc* 1995; **54**: 94A

18 Gris JC, Schved JF, Feugeas O *et al*. Impact of smoking, physical training and weight reduction on factor VII, PAI-1 and haemostatic markers in sedentary men. *Thromb Haemost* 1990; **64**: 516–20

19 Ornish D, Brown SE, Scherlitz B *et al*. Lifestyle changes reverse coronary heart disease. *Lancet* 1990; **336**: 129–33

20 Watts NB, Lewis B, Brunt JNH. Effects on coronary heart disease of a lipid lowering diet, or diet plus cholestyramine. *Lancet* 1992; **339**: 563–9

21 Blumberg VC, Alexander J. Obesity and the heart. In: Bjorntorp P, Brodoff BN (Eds) *Obesity*. Philadelphia: Lippincott, 1992; 517–31

22 Messerli FH. Cardiovascular effects of obesity and hypertension. *Lancet* 1982; **1**: 1165–7

23 Shinton R, Shipley M, Rose G. Overweight and stroke in the Whitehall study. *J Epidemiol Community Health* 1991; **45**: 138–42

24 DiPietro L, Ostfeld AM, Rosner GL. Adiposity and stroke among older adults of low socioeconomic status: the Chicago Stroke Study. *Am J Public Health* 1994; **84**: 14–9

25 Shinton R, Sagar G, Beevers G. Body fat and stroke: unmasking the hazards of overweight and obesity. *J Epidemiol Community Health* 1995; **49**: 259–64

26 Rimm AA, Werner LH, Van Yserloo B, Bernstein RA. Relationship of obesity and disease in 73,532 weight conscious women. *Public Health Rep* 1975; **90**: 44–51

27 Bray GA. Complications of obesity. *Ann Intern Med* 1985; **103**: 1052–61

28 Friedman GD, Kannel WB, Dawber JR. The epidemiology of gallbladder disease: observations from the Framingham study. *J Chronic Dis* 1966; **19**: 273–92

29 Stampfer MJ, Maclure KM, Colditz KM *et al*. Risk of symptomatic gallstones in women with severe obesity. *Am J Clin Nutr* 1992; **55**: 652–8

30 Klain J, Fraser D, Goldstein J *et al*. Liver histology abnormalities in the morbidly obese. *Hepatology* 1989; **10**: 873–6

31 Levi F, La Vecchia C, Negri T *et al*. Body mass at different ages and subsequent endometrial cancer risk. *Int J Cancer* 1992; **50**: 567–71

32 Deslypere JP. Obesity and cancer. *Metabolism* 1995; **44 Suppl 3**: 24–7

33 Tornberg SA, Canstensen J. Relationship between Quetelet's index and cancer of breast and female genital tract in 47,000 women followed for 25 years. *Br J Cancer* 1994; **69**: 358–61

34 Kabat G, Wynden E. Body mass index and lung cancer risk. *Am J Epidemiol* 1992; **135**: 769–74

35 McGoey BB, Deitel M, Saplys RJF, Kliman ME. Effect of weight loss on musculoskeletal pain in the morbidly obese. *J Bone Joint Surg [Br]* 1990; **72**: 322–3

36 Compsten JE, Laskery MA, Croucher PI, Coxon A, Kreitzman ME. Effect of diet induced weight loss on total body bone mass. *Clin Sci* 1992; **82**: 429–32

37 Rissanen A, Heliovaara M, Knect P, Reunanen A, Aromaa A, Maatela J. Risk of diability and mortality due to overweight in a Finnish population. *BMJ* 1990; **301**: 835–7

38 Bjorntorp P. Endocrine abnormalities of obesity. *Metabolism* 1995; **44 Suppl 3**: 21–3

39 Marin P, Kvist H, Lindstedt G *et al*. Low concentrations of insulin-like growth factor 1 in abdominal obesity. *Int J Obes* 1993; **17**: 83–9

40 Jung RT, Campbell RG, James WPT, Callingham BA. Altered hypothalamic and sympathetic responses to hypoglycaemia in familial obesity. *Lancet* 1982; **1**: 1043–6

41 Pasquali R, Cantobelli S, Casimirra F *et al*. The hypothalamic pituitary adrenal axis in obese women with different patterns of body fat distribution. *J Clin Endocrinol Metab* 1993; **77**: 341–6

42 Marin P, Darin N, Amemiya T, Andersson B, Jern S, Bjorntorp P. Cortisol secretion in relation to body fat distribution in obese premenopausal women. *Metabolism* 1992; **41**: 882–6

43 Lapidus L, Bengtsson C, Hallstrom T, Bjorntorp P. Obesity, adipose tissue distribution and health in women. results from a population study in Gothenburg, Sweden. *Appetite* 1989; **12**: 25–35

44 Jayo J, Shively C, Kaplan J *et al*. Effects of exercise and stress on body fat distribution in male cynomologus monkeys. *Int J Obes* 1993; **17**: 597–604

45 Kopelman PG. Altered respiratory function in obesity: sleep disordered breathing and the Pickwickian syndrome. In: Bjorntorp P, Brodoff BN (Eds) *Obesity*. Philadelphia: Lippincott, 1992; 568–75

46   Kalkhoff RK. Obesity in pregnancy. In: Bjorntorp P, Brodoff BN (Eds) *Obesity*. Philadelphia: Lippincott, 1992; 568–75
47   Garbaciak JA, Richter M, Miller S, Barton JJ. Maternal weight and pregnancy complications. *Am J Obstet Gynecol* 1985; **152**: 238–43
48   Edwards LE, Dickes WF, Alton IR, Hakanson EY. Pregnancy in the massively obese: course, outcome, and obesity prognosis of the infant. *Am J Obstet Gynecol* 1978; **131**: 479–83
49   Shaw GM, Velie EM, Schaffer D. Risk of neural tube defect affected pregnancies among obese women. *JAMA* 1996; **275**: 1093–6
50   Wolf AM, Colditz GA. The cost of obesity; the US perspective. *PharmacoEconomics* 1994; **5 Suppl 1**: 34–7

Obesity, non-insulin-dependent diabetes mellitus and the metabolic syndrome

Peter G Kopelman and **Lorraine Albon**

St Bartholomew's and The Royal London School of Medicine and Dentistry, Queen Mary and Westfield College, London, UK

Obesity is characterised by alterations in metabolic function which result from a combination of increasing total body fatness and the regional distribution of adipose tissue. Abdominal visceral obesity is particularly associated with hyperinsulinaemia, increased portal vein free fatty acid concentration, hepatic gluconeogenesis, altered adrenocortical activity and androgen secretion and reduced plasma sex hormone binding globulin levels. These alterations, which are accompanied by changes in visceral adipocyte sensitivity to plasma catecholamine stimulation, enhance further visceral fat deposition and the perpetuation of the metabolic derangements. The characteristic dyslipidaemia associated with upper body obesity and the frequent development of NIDDM are predictable consequences. In contrast to the considerable knowledge about the biochemical background to these alterations, relatively little is understood about the mechanisms through which an individual's ethnic background influences the changes. This chapter reviews these important issues.

Obesity is characterised by altered metabolic function, a consequence of increasing body fatness. The cellular mechanisms involved in these changes, and their relationship to the metabolic aberrations associated with the distribution of adipose tissue, are now better understood. It has become clear that such metabolic alterations may be closely involved with the development of important complications of obesity — ischaemic heart disease and diabetes mellitus. This chapter reviews the alterations of metabolic function seen particularly in subjects with 'upper body' obesity, and describes the likely chain of cellular events which may culminate in the development of dyslipidaemia and diabetes mellitus.

Insulin secretion in obesity

Correspondence to:
Dr Peter Kopelman,
Medical Unit,
Royal London Hospital,
London E1 1BB, UK

Obesity is characterised by an elevated fasting plasma insulin and an exaggerated insulin response to an oral glucose load[1]. Obesity and body fat distribution influence glucose metabolism through independent but additive mechanisms. Kissebah and colleagues[2] have demonstrated that increasing 'upper body' obesity is accompanied by a progressive increase in the glucose and insulin response to an oral glucose challenge. Individuals' *in vivo* insulin sensitivity was assessed further by determining the steady state plasma glucose (SSPG) and insulin (SSPI) attained during a simultaneous intravenous infusion of somatostatin, insulin and dextrose. Since endogenous insulin production was suppressed by somatostatin and the SSPI was comparable in each situation, SSPG directly measured the subjects' ability to dispose of an intravenous glucose load under the same insulin stimulus. SSPG can be taken as an index of insulin resistance. The results showed a positive correlation between increasing upper body obesity and SSPG. After adjustment for the effects of overall fatness (% ideal body weight), upper body obesity remained independently correlated with SSPG suggesting that the location of body fat is an independent factor influencing the degree of insulin sensitivity and, in turn, metabolic profile.

Measurement of portal plasma insulin levels (as an index of insulin secretion) show similar levels in upper body and lower body obesity but hepatic insulin extraction, both basally and during stimulation by intravenous or oral glucose, is reduced in upper body obesity[3]. As a consequence, post hepatic insulin delivery is increased in upper body obesity leading to more marked peripheral insulin concentrations. Studies of insulin sensitivity and responsiveness of skeletal muscle and the relationship to overall glucose disposal in premenopausal women, with varying body fat distribution, have revealed a significant decline as upper body fatness increases[4]. Insulin-stimulated activity of the glucose-6-phosphate independent form of glycogen synthase (GSI) was measured in quadricep muscle biopsies taken during a somatostatin-insulin-dextrose infusion. Despite comparable degrees of SSPI in all women, significant reductions in percentage GSI were seen as the degree of upper body fatness increased and this was accompanied by decreased efficiency in insulin-stimulated glucose disposal (reflected by increasing SSPG at similar SSPI levels). Furthermore, a significant trend was reported for a decreased number of cellular insulin receptors associated with increasing upper body fatness, which was associated in some subjects with reduced glucose disposal during supra-maximal insulin stimulation. Such findings suggest a defect at both the level of the insulin receptor and in post-receptor events.

The possibility that insulin resistance in obesity is either due to a decreased number of insulin-sensitive glucose transporters (GLUT) or an inability to stimulate recruitment of transporters from microsomes to the plasma membrane has been investigated in obese humans. Garvey and colleagues[5] measured GLUT 4 expression in adipocytes — GLUT 4 is the transporter which mediates the bulk of insulin-stimulated transport activity. They found that obesity led to a depletion of intracellular GLUT

4 transporters with fewer carriers being available for insulin-mediated recruitment to the cell surface. The cellular content of GLUT 4 was determined by the GLUT 4 mRNA over a wide range of body weight. In non-insulin dependent diabetic patients (NIDDM), profound insulin resistance was caused by a more severe depletion of GLUT 4 mRNA compared to simple obesity and transporter loss involved both plasma membrane and intracellular compartments[5]. In both obesity and NIDDM, pre-translational suppression of GLUT 4 transporters entirely accounted for impaired cellular insulin responsiveness in adipose tissue. In contrast, no significant differences were seen in skeletal muscle GLUT 4 content and GLUT 4 mRNA activity was similar to that seen control subjects[6]. Other mechanisms which could potentially impair glucose transport activity in skeletal muscle include decreased functional activity of the transporters, or an impairment of insulin-stimulated translocation of intracellular GLUT 4 to the cell surface. It has been demonstrated that chronic exposure to high concentrations of glucose and insulin reduce the subsequent ability of insulin to maximally stimulate glucose transport by inhibiting transporter translocation[7]. The *in vivo* efficacy of skeletal muscle glucose uptake has been shown to be inversely proportional to the glycosylated haemoglobin value in NIDDM subjects[8]. Thus hyperglycaemia and/or hyperinsulinaemia could induce at least a component of insulin resistance in muscle via such mechanisms.

Normal adipose tissue function

Fat tissue mass is dependent on the number and size of adipocytes. Adipocytes have the unique characteristic of being dominated by their contents of storage fats, triglycerides. The mass of triglycerides in an adipocyte is dependent on the balance between triglyceride influx and mobilisation; the latter in the form of free fatty acids (FFA) and glycerol is regulated by metabolic processes under hormonal and nervous system control. Formation of new adipocytes seems to occur when cells reach a certain size and is apparently dependent on various factors, such as age, gender and nutrition[9]. The body fat's stores are almost entirely in the form of triacylglycerol (TAG) in adipocytes. The process of fat mobilisation consists of hydrolysis of the stored TAG to release non-esterified fatty acids (NEFA) into the circulation. The key enzyme is the intracellular TAG-lipase, hormone sensitive lipase (HSL). The major regulator of HSL is reversible phosphorylation by a cAMP-dependent protein kinase. Lipolysis is, therefore, stimulated by effectors which increase the activity of adenylate cyclase in adipocytes leading to the formation of cAMP from ATP. Adenylate cyclase is stimulated by hormones acting via the cell surface receptors and G-proteins, especially catecholamines acting via β-adrenoreceptors (β_1, β_2, β_3)[10-12]. Dephosphorylation of HSL occurs when cAMP concentrations fall. The main hormonal regulator of this is insulin, which lowers adipocyte cAMP concentrations[13]. The suppression of fat mobilisation occurs in normal circumstances at very low insulin concentrations. Catecholamines acting on α_2-adrenoreceptors will also inhibit lipolysis[12,14]. Thus catecholamines have dual effects on the lipolysis rates, both accelerating through β-adrenoceptors and retarding through α_2-adrenoceptors. HSL activity is suppressed after meals when the physiological drive is towards fat storage rather than mobilisation. In the postprandial state, the enzyme lipoprotein lipase (LPL) in adipose tissue is activated by insulin and possibly also by some gastrointestinal peptide hormones[15]. This enzyme is synthesised within adipocytes but exported to the capillary endothelial cells, where it is attached to the luminal side of the capillary wall and acts on circulating TAG in the TAG-rich lipoproteins (chylomicrons and very low density lipoproteins, VLDL). LPL releases fatty acids which may be taken up into the tissue for esterification and storage as TAG. The fatty acids released by LPL action are not all taken up by adipose tissue for storage with approximately 50% entering the systemic circulation[16]. This release of LPL-derived fatty acids is dependent upon the insulin response to the meal and the sensitivity of LPL activation to insulin and other hormones.

Regional distribution of body fat

There is considerable evidence for lipoprotein lipase (LPL) playing a controlling rate in the regional distribution of fat. There are significant gender and regional differences in LPL activity that largely parallel variations in fat size. Premenopausal women have higher LPL activities in gluteal and femoral regions than men but the differences disappear after the menopause[17]. In addition, women have quantitatively more LPL in gluteal and femoral tissue, which contain larger fat cells than they do in abdominal adipose tissue. In contrast, men show minimal regional variations in LPL activity or fat cell size. These differences in fat distribution between men and women may explain the tendency for premenopausal women to deposit fat preferentially in lower body fat depots.

The potential differences in FFA metabolism between lean and obese subjects may reflect the anti-lipolytic effectiveness of insulin in obesity, the relationship of FFA release to the amount of body fat and the lipolytic responsiveness of obese individuals to catecholamines. It is relevant that adipocytes from various body regions differ from one another in many respects; fat cell size and basal lipolysis varying in adipocytes from omental, abdominal subcutaneous and gluteal-thigh depots[18]. The basal release of FFA from adipose tissue to meet lean body mass energy needs is greater in upper body obese women than obese women with lower body fat distribution and non-obese women. Differences in the ability of insulin to suppress lipolysis and of catecholamines to stimulate lipolysis also varies according to fat distribution[19]. In both men and women, the lipolytic response to noradrenaline, which acts via α_2- and β-adrenoceptors, is more marked in abdominal than gluteal or femoral tissues[20]. A detailed analysis has suggested that the usual pattern of male fat distribution (greater abdominal fat accumulation) results from a greater α_2 activity in the abdominal tissue of men[21]. The findings from studies looking at radioligand binding of β-adrenergic antagonists have uniformly shown twice as many β-adrenergic binding sites in abdominal adipocytes as in femoral adipocytes. Lonnqvist and colleagues[22] have recently eluci-dated the pathogenic role of visceral β_3-adrenoceptors in obesity. These authors studied the responsiveness of isolated omental fat cells from obese and non obese subjects to adrenergic-subtype receptor antagonists by measuring the rate of FFA and glycerol response. They found that the visceral fat cells from the obese subjects were highly responsive to noradrenaline stimulation. This appeared mainly due to an enhanced lipolytic response and not to FFA re-utilisation. The main finding was the markedly augmented β_3-adrenoceptor sensitivity and coupling efficiency; the authors suggested that this enhanced β_3-adrenoreceptor activity was due to an increased receptor number in obese subjects. In contrast, the net lipolytic response to adrenaline is reduced in upper obese women compared to lower obese and non-obese women. In order for lower obese women to maintain appropriate FFA availability despite increasing fatness, there must be downregulation of lipolysis to prevent FFA release[19]. Martin and colleagues[18] measured FFA release from the leg, non-leg and splanchnic adipose tissue in obese women of differing body fat distribution. The most significant observation was the contrasting differences in lipolytic activity of splanchnic fat between those obese women with predominantly upper body fat and those lower body obese women. This difference was emphasised by the finding of similar FFA release from leg fat in the two groups. The important metabolic interpretation of these data is the apparently elevated rate of lipolysis in visceral fat cells due largely to increased β_3-activity and, partly to α_2-adrenoceptor activity. As a consequence, more FFA is released into the portal system.

Hormonal influences

The hormonal mechanisms regulating adipose tissue LPL activity are not completely understood. Insulin is permissive for LPL synthesis and glucocorticoids enhance the activity of LPL when added with insulin *in vitro*[23]. Sex steroids have been implicated in the regional distribution of body fat and gender differences are seen in LPL activity most particularly during pregnancy and lactation[24]. Regional variation in receptors for glucocorticoids or sex steroids could play a role in determining regional differences in adipose tissue. The reverse situation may also be true — adipose tissue having an effect on the production of sex hormones. Abdominal visceral adipose tissue is more sensitive to lipolytic stimuli than subcutaneous fat while it is less sensitive to the inhibitory action of insulin; this appears to be associated with a low density of insulin receptors. Hyperinsulinaemia of obesity mainly inhibits lipolysis of insulin sensitive subcutaneous adipocytes and thus may accentuate the fraction of systemic FFA originating from visceral fat[25,26]. In addition, elevated portal concentrations of FFA, produced by active visceral adipocytes, results in the liver being exposed to excessive FFA concentrations. The excessive visceral fat lipolysis may create a vicious chain of events with insulin resistance in liver and skeletal muscle resulting in additional systemic insulin resistance.

Steroid hormones

Obese subjects have a normal circulating plasma cortisol concentration with a normal circadian rhythm and normal urinary free cortisol but an accelerated degradation of cortisol which is compensated by an increased cortisol production rate[27,28]. It is likely that the increase in metabolic clearance of cortisol is secondary to a decrease in cortisol-binding globulin plasma concentrations. Slavnov and colleagues[29] have reported a moderate elevation in plasma corticotrophin (ACTH) levels in obesity to explain the increased cortisol production. The increased peripheral clearance rate of cortisol is probably mediated by binding to the glucocorticoid receptor present in glucocorticoid responding tissue[30]. An increased peripheral density of this receptor will be followed by an increased metabolic clearance rate. Cortisol has effects on both lipid accumulation and mobilisation. Cortisol inhibits the anti-lipolytic effect of insulin in human adipocytes and this may be particularly pronounced in visceral abdominal fat[23]. It also has a permissive effect on lipid mobilisation stimulated by catecholamine. Enlarged visceral adipocytes, as found in abdominal obesity, could be the site where this occurs because such tissue appears to have a higher density of glucocorticoid receptors compared to adipose tissue[31,32]. Abdominal subcutaneous adipose tissue demonstrates a higher expression of cortisol-induced LPL as well as a higher density of glucocorticoid receptors than femoral subcutaneous adipose tissue. Furthermore, there is a higher LPL activity in visceral compared to subcutaneous adipose tissue in both men and women[33]. This could be an explanation for the functional hypercortisolism associated with abdominal obesity in subjects who are only moderately overweight. There is a close analogy between upper body obesity and Cushing's syndrome because both conditions are characterised by hypercortisolism and excessive visceral fat accumulation[34]. Moreover, both have similar consequences — increasing plasma cortisol leading to insulin insensitivity and glucose intolerance, an increase in hepatic gluconeogenesis, reduced hepatic insulin uptake and insulin resistance in skeletal muscle.

The increased peripheral clearance and the obesity-associated acceleration in overall adrenocortical function leads also to an increase in adrenal androgen production. Urinary 17-ketosteroids (17-KS), which measure various androgen metabolites including etiocholananolone, androsterone, dehydroepiandrosterone (DHEA), and its sulphate conjugate (DHEAS), are elevated in obese subjects[35]. The changes in adrenal androgen production may simply occur in compensation for an increasing metabolic clearance, but there is additional evidence to suggest alterations in adrenocortical dynamics. Kurtz and colleagues[36] noted an increased turnover of DHEA in obese women. These authors demonstrated a significant correlation between upper body obesity and the metabolic clearance of DHEA and androstenedione, which suggests that the androgenic effects of DHEA may have a role in fat distribution. In premenopausal women, serum DHEA concentration correlates positively with trunk fat and negatively with leg fat accumulation, whereas no such effect is seen in men[37,38]. A shift in fat accumulation in women towards abdominal obesity may be an androgenic effect of DHEA. In healthy postmenopausal women, androgen levels are inversely related to fasting plasma glucose levels and are predictive of central obesity 10–15 years later[39]. Brody *et al.*[40] have reported a positive correlation between body weight and changes in DHEA and the DHEA/17-hydroxy progesterone ratio after exogenous administration of ACTH. This is suggestive of hyper-responsiveness of adrenal androgens in obesity. Weaver and colleagues[41] have also provided evidence for increased ACTH release in obesity by reporting an association between the ACTH response to insulin-induced hypoglycaemia and increasing body weight. Moreover, alterations in adrenocortical production of adrenal androgens probably reflects the influence of other factors, including adrenal androgens themselves. *In vitro* studies have suggested a lesser degree of inhibition of human 17-hydroxylase activity by DHEA as compared to the inhibition of human 17,20-desmolase activity[42]. The increased adipose tissue breakdown and the higher urinary excretion of DHEA in such circumstances could lead to decreased intra-adrenal concentrations of the steroid. As a consequence, the inhibition of 17,20-desmolase will be further diminished and a selective increase in the production of DHEA and its metabolites occur.

DHEA may, therefore, contribute to a spiral of events — the greater androgenic action of DHEA contributing to abdominal fat cell accumulation with resulting hyperglycaemia and hyperinsulinaemia. Androgens have a clear effect on adipose tissue metabolism; this includes enhancement of lipolytic sensitivity by expression of lipolytic β-adrenergic receptors via an androgenic receptor, which is positively autoregulated by testosterone[43,44].

The density of androgen receptors, which are specific for androgens, varies in different adipose tissue regions with a higher density in intra-abdominal than subcutaneous depots in rats[45]. Indirect evidence suggests a higher density in central visceral fat in man compared to peripheral adipose tissue[25]. Testosterone, in the presence of growth hormone (GH), exerts a dramatic effect on the regulation of lipolysis by increasing the number of β-adrenoceptors through an action at the level of adenylate cyclase and protein kinase A and/or HSL[43,44,46].

Sex steroid secretion

There appear to be contrasting situations between men and women in relation to the influence of sex steroids on adipose tissue function. Men, with excessive abdominal fat, often have relatively low serum testosterone concentrations despite reduced levels of sex hormone binding globulin (SHBG)[47]. Marin and colleagues[48] have demonstrated a significant decrease in visceral fat mass and abdominal:sagittal diameter in middle aged abdominally obese men treated with 8 months of oral testosterone supplements. This reduction occurred without a detectable change in subcutaneous fat. In addition, there was an improvement in plasma glucose disposal and increased insulin sensitivity. The authors concluded that such men have relative hypogonadism and associated metabolic abnormalities, which are partly corrected by testosterone supplementation. Calculations of lipid uptake and LPL activity, using isotope labelling techniques, suggested diminished activity in abdominal adipose tissue but no change in femoral fat[49,50]. The effects of testosterone were much more marked in visceral fat compared to subcutaneous abdominal fat because the uptake of lipid was inhibited by approximately 50% in the intra-abdominal tissues. This has been confirmed by studies of lipid turnover in visceral adipose tissue from rats. Thus, testosterone supplementation in obese men decreases uptake of lipid particularly in visceral fat and increases the rate of fat mobilisation.

Obese women are also characterised by distinct alterations in circulating sex hormone levels[51]. Obese women demonstrate lower circulating SHBG levels and, thereby, an increased fraction of circulating oestradiol. In postmenopausal obese women, serum levels of oestrone and oestradiol are correlated with the degree of obesity and fat mass[52]. The plasma ratio of oestrone to oestradiol is also increased in obesity. Interestingly, a similar pattern of changes of sex steroid concentrations and binding are found in women with the polycystic ovary syndrome[53]. Longcope and colleagues[54] have reported significant associations between body weight and conversion of testosterone to oestradiol. The interconversion of oestrone to oestradiol has been observed *in vivo* and *in vitro* in adipose tissue with a greater conversion being found in omental fat than subcutaneous fat[55,56]. Adipose tissue 17-β-hydroxysteroid dehydrogenase activity, measured by the conversion of oestrone to oestradiol, is higher in premenopausal than in postmenopausal women and all women have a higher activity compared to men[56,57].

Evans and colleague[58] have shown that body weight and increasing upper body obesity in women are inversely correlated with SHBG levels and directly correlated to free testosterone concentrations. Others have described a higher production rate from the adrenal cortex and ovaries and increased metabolic clearance of testosterone and dihydrotestosterone (DHT)[51]. The clearance of testosterone increases as SHBG decreases, the consequence of an increased fraction of unbound testosterone available for hepatic extraction and clearance[59]. Such a mechanism may protect some obese women from the development of frank hirsutism. Fat tissue is able to sequester various steroids, including androgens, probably as a result of their lipid solubility. Most sex steroids appear to be preferentially concentrated within adipocytes rather than in the plasma[60]. As a result, the overall steroid pool in severely obese subjects is far greater than that of normal weight individuals — the volume of fat in obese subjects is much larger than the intravascular space and tissue steroid concentration is 2–13 times higher than in plasma. Fat may serve not only as a reservoir but also as a site for steroid metabolism. Androgens can be irreversibly aromatised to oestrogens or reversibly converted to other androgens[61–63]. Peripheral aromatisation increases with age and is 2–4 times higher in postmenopausal women[64]. Androstenedione is the major substrate for peripheral oestrogen formation. In contrast, only a small amount of testosterone is converted to oestradiol, although this may be of greater clinical significance.

The androgen receptor in adipose tissue from women seems to have the same specificity and affinity as in men suggesting the receptor is identical. 17-β oestradiol appears to decrease androgen receptor density because oophorectomy is necessary for testosterone to result in an increase in visceral fat mass in a woman[65]. It seems possible that oestrogen protects from the androgen effects by down-regulation of androgen receptors[66]. The centralisation of body fat after the menopause, leading to a male type of adipose tissue, could be due to the loss of this protective effects of oestrogen from androgens by allowing the expression of more androgen receptors. It is of interest that hyperandrogenic women have body fat distribution which resembles males[67]. Oestrogen replacement in postmenopausal women leads to a marked elevation of LPL activity specifically in the gluteo-femoral region, which results in a similar metabolic pattern of activity of adipose tissue from this region compared to that seen in pre-menopausal women[66,68]. No specific hormonal receptors have been identified for oestrogen and progesterone and these effects may be mediated through competition with glucocorticoid receptors thereby protecting against the effects of cortisol, possibly by downregulation of the receptor[69].

Sex hormone binding globulin in obesity

SHBG is a circulating globulin produced by the liver which binds in high affinity, but low capacity, to many of the circulating sex hormones[70]. Alterations in SHBG levels have a profound impact on the metabolism and action of bound steroids. A decrease of SHBG concentration is associated with an increase in metabolic clearance and free fraction of testosterone and oestradiol. The hypothesis that insulin may regulate the hepatic production of SHBG is supported by the finding of a direct inhibitory action of insulin on SHBG secretion by cultured human hepatoma cells[71]. Peiris and colleagues[72] have shown upper body obesity in women to be associated with increased pancreatic insulin production and decreased hepatic insulin clearance. Thus, increasing splanchnic insulin concentrations may account for decreased hepatic SHBG production in this type of obesity. These authors also showed the severity of the peripheral insulin resistance to be positively correlated with the magnitude of free testosterone — the greater the free testosterone level, the greater the degree of insulin resistance. The changes in circulating androgens do not appear to influence plasma insulin levels but, conversely, increasing plasma insulin may increase androgen secretion by a number of mechanisms which include direct stimulation of androgen production by the ovary[73]. There is recent evidence to suggest that both insulin and insulin-like growth factor 1 (IGF-1) may be important regulators of ovarian thecal and stromal androgen production with an interaction at the receptor level on the ovarian stroma of these two hormones[74].

Dyslipidaemia and upper body obesity

Hyperinsulinaemia and insulin resistance are both significant correlates of a dyslipoproteinaemic state which is characteristic of upper body obesity. The lipolysis of insulin resistant visceral adipocytes results in predictable and characteristic changes. These are reflected by an elevated fasting plasma triglyceride concentration, reduced HDL-cholesterol, marginal elevations of cholesterol and LDL-cholesterol concentrations and increased number of apo-B carrying lipoproteins[75,76]. Measurement of the volume of visceral fat, using computerised tomography (CT) scanning, confirms a close relationship between the volume of visceral adipose tissue, elevation of plasma triglyceride and decreased concentration of HDL and HDL_2-cholesterol in both men and women[77]. Moreover, these levels are comparable in men and women when matched for similar degrees of visceral adiposity[78].

The elevated plasma NEFA concentrations have a number of deleterious actions: plasma NEFAs are the major substrate for hepatic TAG synthesis and there is a close correlation between NEFA and VLDL-TAG concentrations or turnover rates[79]. This increased turnover appears to alter the balance between intracellular degradation of newly synthesised hepatic lipoprotein-B (apo-B) and its secretion as VLDL. The increased availability of NEFA not only increases VLDL-TAG secretion but also the number of VLDL particles secreted[80]. This may be particularly important in the postprandial period.

Insulin has an acute suppressive action on both NEFA supply to the liver and hepatic VLDL secretion in the postprandial period. In cultured hepatocytes, insulin inhibits VLDL secretion[81]. This action reduces the competition for clearance and reduces the postprandial rise in TAG concentration. A failure to normally suppress the NEFA supply, seen in subjects with increased intra-abdominal fat tissue, will lead to a sustained production of VLDL and an impaired clearance of TAG-rich lipoproteins in the postprandial period[9]. Plasma NEFA arise in the postprandial period both from intracellular lipolysis and from the action of LPL in capillaries. A failure of the entrapment of fatty acids in adipose tissue during the action of LPL on chylomicron-TAG may be an important mechanism leading to increased VLDL secretion[80]. A further consequence is an increase of LDL particles — VLDL is a precursor of

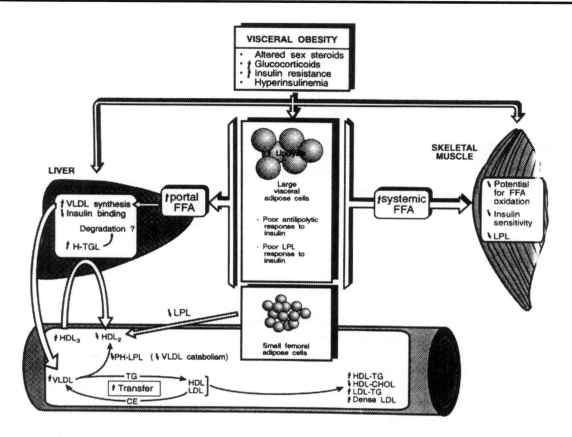

Fig. 1 A schematic outline of the alterations observed in plasma lipid transport and lipoprotein metabolism associated with abdominal visceral obesity. Alterations in adrenocortical function (including sex steroids) and plasma insulin concentrations create a chain of events illustrated in the diagram. Enlargement of visceral adipocytes is accompanied by increased free fatty acid (FFA) in the portal and systemic circulation which results in increased triglyceride synthesis and VLDL secretion. This, in turn, may contribute to the prevailing hyperinsulinaemia. The slower catabolism of triglyceride–rich lipoproteins due to reduced lipoprotein lipase (LPL) activity, in skeletal muscle and adipose tissue, may explain the reduced HDL–cholesterol levels in visceral obesity. Hepatic–triglyceride lipase (H–TGL) activity is increased which also leads to reduced HDL–cholesterol levels. Elevated triglyceride levels favour the transfer of lipids among lipoproteins resulting in triglyceride enrichment of HDL and LDL while VLDL are enriched in cholesterol esters (CE). The small triglyceride–rich LDL and HDL particles are good substrates for H–TGL and this leads to the formation of dense LDL particles. Elevated plasma concentrations of dense LDL particles are associated with the development of coronary heart disease. Reproduced from Despres[78] with kind permission of the author and the editors of *Baillière's Clinical Endocrinology and Metabolism.*

LDL — but not necessarily an increase in LDL-cholesterol concentration since, in the presence of high VLDL-TAG concentrations, LDL particles are lipid depleted and thus more dense. An elevation of total plasma apo-B concentration is a frequent association with upper body obesity which, by itself, heightens the risk of coronary heart disease[82].

Other factors which contribute to the dyslipoproteinaemia in upper body obesity include increased sex steroid and glucocorticoid: glucocorticoids stimulate VLDL and apo-B production, decrease the activity of the LDL receptor and contribute to the insulin resistant state[83]. Figure 1 summarises the alterations in plasma lipid transport and lipoprotein metabolism seen in viscerally obese subjects.

From obesity to NIDDM

The deleterious metabolic effects of altered regulation of adipocyte function, observed particularly in visceral obesity, frequently leads to the development of impaired glucose tolerance and NIDDM.

In obesity, the rate of non-esterified fatty acid (NEFA) turnover/unit lean body mass is increased[84]. The ability of insulin to suppress NEFA release *in vivo* is diminished in obese subjects as a result of alterations in insulin sensitivity of both lipolytic processes and fatty acid re-esterification. It is, therefore, unsurprising that plasma NEFA increases when insulin action is deficient (as in NIDDM)[84,85]. A cycle of events is thereby entered with increasing insulin resistance resulting in increasing NEFA plasma concentration which, in turn, contributes to diminishing insulin sensitivity. The defect in insulin sensitivity observed in skeletal muscle may accentuate the defects in the regulation of lipolysis.

A number of mechanisms link NEFA supply and impairment of glucose utilisation with the supply of NEFA to the liver being an important determinant of the rate of hepatic glucose production. The elevation in plasma NEFA concentration, particularly postprandially when they are usually suppressed, will lead to an inappropriate maintenance of glucose production and an impairment of glucose utilisation (impaired glucose tolerance). These mechanisms may be critical links leading from obesity to the development of NIDDM. The progression to NIDDM may be enhanced by the suppressive effects of high NEFA concentrations on insulin secretion or even by potentially 'toxic' effects of NEFA on pancreatic β cells[86]. A further mechanism linking increased plasma NEFA concentrations to insulin resistance is the reduced hepatic clearance of insulin — increasing delivery of NEFA to the liver reduces insulin binding to the hepatocytes. In normal circumstances, the liver removes 40% of insulin secreted from the pancreas; an impairment of this process will have a significant effect on peripheral (systemic) insulin concentrations, which contributes to hyperinsulinaemia, and leads to further down-regulation of insulin receptors and increasing insulin resistance[87].

In the initial phases of this process, the pancreas can respond by maintaining a state of compensatory hyperinsulinaemia with gross decompensation of glucose tolerance being prevented. With ever increasing plasma concentrations of NEFA, the insulin resistant individual cannot continue to maintain this state of compensatory hyperinsulinaemia, and hyperglycaemia prevails in time. Thus, increasing NEFA concentrations, associated with a small decline in insulin secretion, will further decrease glucose uptake by muscle, increase hepatic NEFA oxidation and stimulate gluconeogenesis. This has an additive effect on plasma elevations of NEFA and glucose which, in turn, further compromises β cell function[88].

The effect of weight reduction

The beneficial action of weight reduction suggests that many, if not all, of the deleterious events associated with upper body obesity are a consequence, rather than a cause, of excessive visceral adipose tissue.

Weight reduction in women with upper body obesity has a marked effect on the regulation of lipolysis. There is approximately a 5-fold increase in the sensitivity to noradrenaline with a specific effect on adrenoreceptor subtype — there is increased sensitivity to β_2-receptors but no change in β_1 or α_2. However, no change occurs in the numbers of β_2 receptor binding sites which suggests possible facilitation of G proteins[89]. More recently, a similar pattern of increased sensitivity has been reported for β_3-adrenoreceptors[22]. Weight loss is accompanied by a decrease in circulating insulin levels and a fall in plasma noradrenaline. The beneficial effects of these changes are a decrease in basal lipolysis (with decreased HSL function) and an increase in sensitivity to catecholamine stimulation of lipolysis. Thus weight reduction appears to restore a more efficient regulation of lipolysis with less FFA being released at rest and lower catecholamine levels required for lipolysis activation.

The possible influence of ethnicity on adipocyte distribution and function

Epidemiological studies have identified ethnic difference in both total adiposity and adipocyte distribution. Differences can be demonstrated between nationalities and also within differing ethnic populations in one country. Kertzman and colleagues[90] have identified higher levels of upper body obesity in Israelis from European backgrounds compared to those of other ethnic backgrounds. This difference is maintained despite correction for sporting activity, cigarette smoking and education. Differences have also been shown in body composition between

Polynesians and Caucasians: Polynesians are significantly leaner than Caucasians for any given body size[91].

Such differences in overall body size and fat distribution have implications for health. Some populations appear more at risk than others from visceral adiposity and the concomitant metabolic derangement. South Indians living in the UK have a higher mortality from heart disease than Europeans. Studies have demonstrated higher mean waist hip ratios and trunk skinfold thickness in South Asians compared to Europeans of similar body weight[92]. The South Asian group are also characterised by higher blood pressures, higher fasting and post oral glucose insulin levels, higher triglyceride and lower HDL cholesterol. These results suggest that South Asians are particularly prone to the development of upper body obesity and the associated derangements of metabolic function[93]. In contrast, subjects of Afro-Caribbean origin have a low mortality rate from coronary heart disease in spite of a high prevalence of diabetes[94]. Glucose intolerance in Afro-Caribbean subjects is twice as common compared to Europeans, while the prevalence of probable heart disease in Afro-Caribbean men is approximately half that seen in European males. Interestingly, Afro-Caribbean men generally have less abdominal adiposity compared to Europeans and this seems to confer an advantageous lipid profile. It is speculated that the favourable lipoprotein profile, which persists despite glucose intolerance, is related to body fat distribution in Afro-Caribbeans and explains the lower levels of cardiac mortality.

There is little published work addressing possible differences in adipocyte function between subjects from different ethnic backgrounds. An investigation of the ability of insulin to stimulate glucose transport and suppress lipolysis, suggests that ethnicity is important[95]. In this study, abdominal and gluteal adipocytes from white women with upper body obesity were less sensitive, *in vitro*, to insulin stimulated glucose transport and lipolytic suppression compared to adipocytes from black women of similar body weight and fat distribution. The findings support the epidemiological evidence that black women, with upper body obesity, fare better in terms of insulin resistance and dyslipidaemia than their white counterparts and confirm the need for additional studies examining men and women from other ethic groups.

References

1   Kolterman OG, Insel J, Sackow M, Olefsky M. Mechanisms of insulin resistance in human obesity. *J Clin Invest* 1980; **65**: 1272–84

2   Kissebah AH, Vydelingum N, Murray R. Relation of body fat distribution to metabolic complications of obesity. *J Clin Invest* 1982; **54**: 254–60

3   Peiris AN, Mueller RA, Smith GA. Splanchnic insulin metabolism in obesity: influence of body fat distribution. *J Clin Invest* 1986; **78**: 1648–57

4   Evans DJ, Murray R, Kissebah AH. Relationship between skeletal muscle insulin resistance, insulin-mediated glucose disposal and insulin binding effects of obesity and body fat topography. *J Clin Invest* 1984; **74**: 1515–25

5   Garvey WT, Maianu L, Huecksteadt TP *et al.* Pretranslational suppression of a glucose transporter protein causes cellular insulin resistance in non-insulin dependent diabetes and obesity. *J Clin Invest* 1991; **87**: 1072–81

6   Garvey WT, Maianu L, Hancock JA, Golichowski AM, Baron A. Gene expression of GLUT 4 in skeletal muscle from insulin-resistant patients with obesity, IGT, GDM, NIDDM. *Diabetes* 1992; **41**: 465–75

7   Garvey WT, Olefsky JM, Matthaei S, Marshall S. Glucose and insulin coregulate the glucose transport system in primary cultured adipocytes: a new mechanism of insulin resistance. *J Biol Chem* 1987; **262**: 189–97

8   Baron A, Laakso M, Brechtel G, Edelman SV. Reduced capacity and affinity of skeletal muscle for insulin-mediated glucose uptake in non-insulin dependent diabetic subjects. *J Clin Invest* 1991; **87**: 1186–94

9   Frayn B, Williams CM, Arner P. Are increased plasma non-esterified fatty acid concentrations a risk marker for coronary heart disease and other chronic diseases? *Clin Sci* 1996; **90**: 243–53

10   Wahrenberg H, Lonnqvist F, Arner P. Mechanisms underlying regional differences in lipolysis in human adipose tissue. *J Clin Invest* 1989; **84**: 458–67

11   Burns TW, Langley PE. Lipolysis by human adipose tissue: the role of cyclic 3′,5′-adenosine monophosphate and adrenergic receptors. *J Lab Clin Med* 1970; **75**: 983–7

12   Lafontan M, Berlan M. Fat cell adrenergic receptors and the control of white and brown fat cell function. *J Lipid Res* 1993; **34**: 1057–91

13   Smith CJ, Vasta V, Degerman E, Belfrage P, Manganiello VC. Hormone-sensitive cyclic GMP-inhibited cyclic AMP phosphodiesterase in rat adipocytes. Regulation of insulin- and cAMP-dependent activation by phosphorylation. *J Biol Chem* 1991; **266**: 13385–90

14   Castan I, Valet P, Quideau N *et al.* Antilipolytic effects of α_2-agonists, neuropeptide Y, adenosine, and PGE$_1$ in mammal adipocytes. *Am J Physiol* 1994; **266**: R1141–R1147

15   Ong JM, Kern PA. Effect of feeding and obesity on lipoprotein lipase activity, immunoreactive protein and messenger RNA levels in human adipose tissue. *J Clin Invest* 1989; **84**: 305–11

16   Eaton RP, Berman M, Steinberg D. Kinetic studies of plasma free fatty acid and triglyceride metabolism in man. *J Clin Invest* 1969; **48**: 1560–79

17   Rebuffe-Scrive M, Bjorntorp P. Regional adipose tissue metabolism in man. In: Vague J, Bjorntorp P, Guy-Grand B (Eds) *Metabolic Complications of Human Obesities*. Amsterdam: Excerpta Medica, 1985; 149–59

18   Martin ML, Jensen MD. Effects of body fat distribution on regional lipolysis in obesity. *J Clin Invest* 1991; **88**: 609–13

19   Reynisdottir S, Ellerfeldt K, Wahrenberg H, Lithell H, Arner P. Multiple lipolysis defects in insulin resistance (metabolic) syndrome. *J Clin Invest* 1994; **93**: 2590–9

20   Krotkiewski M, Bjorntorp P, Sjostrom L, Smith U. Impact of obesity on metabolism in men and women: importance of regional adipose tissue distribution. *J Clin Invest* 1983; **72**: 1150–62

21   La Fontan M, Dang-Tran L, Berlan M. Alpha-adrenergic antilipolytic effect of adrenaline in human fat cells of the thigh: comparison with adrenal responsiveness of different fat deposits. *Eur J Clin Invest* 1975; **9**: 261–6

22   Lonnqvist F, Thorne A, Nilsell K, Hoffstedt J, Arner P. A pathogenic role of visceral fat β_3-adrenoceptors in obesity. *J Clin Invest* 1995; **95**: 1109–16

23   Cigolini M, Smith U. Human adipose tissue in culture. VIII. Studies on the insulin-antagonistic effect of glucocorticoids. *Metabolism* 1979; **28**: 502–10

24   Rebuffe-Scrive M, Enk L, Crona N *et al.* Fat cell metabolism in different regions in women. Effects of menstrual cycle, pregnancy and lactation. *J Clin Invest* 1985; **75**: 1973–6

25   Rebuffe-Scrive M, Andersson B, Olbe L, Bjorntorp P. Metabolism of adipose tissue in intraabdominal depots of non-obese men and women. *Metabolism* 1989; **38**: 453–61

26   Rebuffe-Scrive M, Krotkiewski M, Elfverson J, Bjorntorp P. Muscle and adipose tissue morphology and metabolism in Cushing's syndrome. *J Clin Endocrinol Metab* 1988; **67**: 1122–8

27 Migeon CJ, Green OC, Eckert JP. Study of adrenocortical function in obesity. *Metabolism* 1963; **12**: 718–30

28 Galvao-Tales A, Graves L, Burke CW *et al*. Free cortisol in obesity: effect of fasting. *Acta Endocrinol* 1976; **81**: 321–9

29 Slavnov VN, Epshtein EV. Somatotrophic, thyrotrophic and adrenotrophic functions of the anterior pituitary in obesity. *Endocrinologie* 1977; **15**: 213–8

30 Rebuffe-Scrive M, Bronnegard M, Nilsso A *et al*. Steroid hormone receptors in human adipose tissues. *J Clin Endocrinol Metab* 1990; **71**: 1215–9

31 Bronnegard M, Arner P, Hellstrom L *et al*. Glucocorticoid receptor messenger ribonucleic acid in different regions of human adipose tissue. *Endocrinology* 1990; **127**: 1689–96

32 Rebuffe-Scrive M, Lundholm K, Bjorntorp P. Glucocorticoid hormone binding to human adipose tissue. *Eur J Clin Invest* 1985; **15**: 267–71

33 Bjorntorp P, Ottosson M, Rebuffe-Scrive M, Xu X. Regional obesity and steroid hormone interactions in human adipose tissue. *UCLA Symp Cell Biol* 1990; **132**: 147–58

34 Mayo-Smith W, Hayes CW, Biller BMK. Body fat distribution measured with CT: correlations in healthy subjects, anorexia nervosa and patients with Cushing's syndrome. *Radiology* 1989; **170**: 515–8

35 Simkin V. Urinary 17-ketosteroid and 17-ketogenic steroid excretion in obese patients. *N Engl J Med* 1961; **264**: 974–7

36 Kurtz BR, Givens JR, Kominder S *et al*. Maintenance of normal circulating levels of androstenedione and dehydroepiandrosterone in simple obesity despite increased metabolic clearance rates: evidence for a servo-controlled mechanism. *J Clin Endocrinol Metab* 1987; **64**: 1261–7

37 Williams DP, Boyden TW, Pamenter RW *et al*. Relationship of body fat percentage and fat distribution with dehydroepiandrosterone sulphate in premenopausal females. *J Clin Endocrinol Metab* 1993; **77**: 80–5

38 Usiskin KS, Butterworth S, Clore JN *et al*. Lack of effect of dehydroepiandrosterone sulphate in obese men. *Int J Obes* 1990; **14**: 457–63

39 Khaw K-T, Barret-Connor E. Fasting plasma glucose levels and endogenous androgens in non-diabetic postmenopausal women. *Clin Sci* 1991; **80**: 199–203

40 Brody S, Carlstrom K, Lagrelius A *et al*. Adrenal steroids in post-menopausal women: relation to obesity and bone mineral content. *Maturitas* 1987; **9**: 25–32

41 Weaver JU, Kopelman PG, McLoughlin L *et al*. Hyperactivity of the hypothalamo-pituitary-adrenal axis in obesity: a study of ACTH, AVP, β-lipoprotein and cortisol responses to insulin-induced hypoglycaemia. *Clin Endocrinol* 1993; **39**: 345–50

42 Couch RM, Muller J, Winter JSD. Regulation of the activities of 17-hydroxylase and 17,20 desmolase in the human adrenal cortex: genetic analysis and inhibition by endogenous steroids. *J Clin Endocrinol Metab* 1986; **63**: 613–8

43 Xu X, De Pergola G, Bjorntorp P. The effects of androgens on the regulation of lipolysis in adipose precursor cells. *Endocrinology* 1990; **126**: 1229–34

44 Xu X, De Pergola G, Bjorntorp P. Testosterone increases lipolysis and the number of β-adrenoceptors in male rat adipocytes. *Endocrinology* 1991; **128**: 379–82

45 Sjogren J, Li M, Bjorntorp P. Androgen hormone binding to adipose tissue in rats. *Biochim Biophys Acta* 1995; **1244**: 117–20

46 Evans BA, Hughes IA. Augmentation of androgen-receptor binding *in vitro*: studies in normals and patients with androgen insensitivity. *Clin Endocrinol* 1985; **23**: 567–77

47 Bjorntorp P. The regulation of adipose tissue distribution in humans. *Int J Obes* 1996; **20**: 291–302

48 Marin P, Holmang S, Jonsson *et al*. The effects of testosterone treatment on body composition and metabolism in middle-aged obese men. *Int J Obes* 1992; **16**: 991–7

49 Marin P, Oden B, Bjorntorp P. Assimilation and mobilization of triglycerides in subcutaneous abdominal and femoral adipose tissue *in vivo* in men: effects of androgens. *J Clin Endocrinol Metab* 1995; **80**: 239–43

50 Marin P, Lonn L, Andersson B *et al*. Assimilation and mobilisation of triglycerides in subcutaneous and intraabdominal adipose tissue *in vivo* in men: effects of testosterone. *J Clin Endocrinol Metab* 1995; **80**: 239–43

51   Kopelman PG. Hormones and obesity. *Baillière's Clin Endocrinol Metab* 1994; **8**: 549–75
52   Meldrum DR, Davidson BJ, Tatryn IV, Judd HL. Changes in circulating steroids with aging in post-menopausal women. *Obstet Gynecol* 1981; **57**: 624–8
53   Baird DT. Polycystic ovary syndrome. In: Jacobs HS (Ed) *Advances in Gynaecological Endocrinology*. London: Proceedings of the Sixth Study Group of the Royal College of Obstetricians and Gynaecologists, 1978; 289–300
54   Longcope C, Baker R, Johnston Jr CC. Androgen and oestrogen metabolism: relationship to obesity. *Metabolism* 1986; **35**: 235–7
55   Longcope C, Layne DS, Tait JF. Metabolic clearance rates and interconversions of oestrone and 17-β-oestradiol in normal males and females. *J Clin Invest* 1986; **47**: 93–106
56   Deslypere JP, Verdonek L, Vermuulen A. Fat tissue: a steroid reservoir and site of steroid metabolism. *J Clin Endocrinol Metab* 1987; **61**: 564–70
57   Roncari DAK, Van RLR. Promotion of human adipocyte precursor replication in 17-β-oestradiol in culture. *J Clin Invest* 1977; **62**: 502–8
58   Evans DJ, Hoffman RG, Kalkhoff R, Kissebah AH. Relationship of androgenic activity of body fat topography, fat cell morphology and metabolic aberrations pre-menopausal women. *J Clin Endocrinol Metab* 1983; **57**: 304–10
59   Vermulen A, Ando S. Metabolic clearance rate and interconversion of androgens and the influence of the free androgen fractions. *J Clin Endocrinol Metab* 1979; **48**: 320–6
60   Feher T, Brodrogi L. A comparative study of steroid concentrations in human adipose tissue and peripheral circulation. *Clin Chim Acta* 1982; **126**: 135–41
61   Longcope C, Kato T, Horton R. Conversion of blood androgens to oestrogens in normal adult men and women. *J Clin Invest* 1969; **48**: 2191–201
62   Schinder AE, Ebert A, Friedrich E. Conversion of androstenedione to oestrone by human fat tissue. *J Clin Endocrinol Metab* 1972; **35**: 627–30
63   Ackerman GE, Smith AE, Mendelson CR *et al*. Aromatization of androstenedione by human adipose tissue stromal cells in monolayer culture. *J Clin Endocrinol Metab* 1981; **53**: 412–7
64   Hemsell DL, Grodin JM, Brenner PF *et al*. Plasma precursors of oestrogen. II. Correlation of the extent of conversion of plasma androstenedione to oestrone with age. *J Clin Endocrinol Metab* 1974; **38**: 476–9
65   Elbers JMH, Asscheman H, Seidell B, Gooren LJG. Increased accumulation of visceral fat after long term androgen administration in women [abstract]. *Int J Obes* 1995; **19 (Suppl 2)**: 25
66   Haarbo J, Marslew U, Gottfredsen A, Christiansen C. Postmenopausal hormone replacement therapy prevents central distribution of body fat after the menopause. *Metabolism* 1991; **40**: 323–6
67   Haffner SM, Katz MS, Stern MP, Dunn JF. The relationship of sex hormones to hyperinsulinaemia and hyperglycaemia. *Metabolism* 1988; **37**: 683–8
68   Rebuffe-Scrive M, Lonnroth P, Marin P, Wesslau C, Bjorntorp P, Smith U. Regional adipose tissue metabolism in men and postmenopausal women. *Int J Obes* 1987; **11**: 347–55
69   Xu X, Hoebeke J, Bjorntorp P. Progestin binds to the glucocorticoid receptor and mediates antiglucocorticoid effect in rat adipose precursor cells. *J Steroid Biochem* 1990; **36**: 465–71
70   Anderson DC. Sex hormone binding globulin. *Clin Endocrinol* 1974; **3**: 69–96
71   Plymate SR, Matej LA, Jones RA, Friedl KE. Inhibition of sex hormone binding globulin production in human hepatoma (hep G2) cell line by insulin and prolactin. *J Clin Endocrinol Metab* 1988; **67**: 460–4
72   Peiris AN, Mueller RA, Strieve MF *et al*. Relationship of androgenic activity to splanchnic insulin metabolism and peripheral glucose utilisation in premenopausal women. *J Clin Endocrinol Metab* 1987; **64**: 162–9
73   Barbieri RL, Hornstein MD. Hyperinsulinaemia and ovarian hyperandrogenism: cause and effect. *Endocrinol Metab Clin North Am* 1988; **17**: 685–703
74   Barbieri RL, Makris A, Randall RW *et al*. Insulin stimulates androgen accumulation in incubations of ovarian stroma obtained from women with hyperandrogenism. *J Clin Endocrinol Metab* 1986; **62**: 904–10
75   Laws A, Reaven GM. Evidence for an independent relationship between insulin resistance and fasting plasma HDL-cholesterol, triglyceride and insulin concentrations. *J Intern Med* 1992; **231**: 25–30

76   Kissebah AH, Peiris AN. Biology of regional body fat distribution: relationship to non-insulin-dependent diabetes mellitus. *Diabetes Metab Rev* 1989; **5**: 83–109

77   Pouliot MC, Despres JP, Nadeau A *et al.* Visceral obesity in men. Associations with glucose tolerance, plasma insulin and lipoprotein levels. *Diabetes* 1992; **41**: 826–34

78   Despres JP. Dyslipidaemia and obesity. *Baillière's Clin Endocrinol Metab* 1994; **8**: 629–60

79   Byrne CD, Brindle NPJ, Wang TWM, Hales CN. Interaction of non-esterified fatty acid and insulin control of triacylglycerol secretion by Hep G2 cells. *Biochem J* 1991; **280**: 99–104

80   Sniderman A, Cainflone K. Metabolic disruptions in the adipocyte-hepatocyte fatty acid axis as the cause of HyperapoB. *Int J Obes* 1995; **19 (Suppl 1)**: S27–S33

81   Durrington PN, Newton RS, Weinstein DB, Steinberg D. Effects of insulin and glucose on very low density lipoprotein triglyceride secretion by cultured rat hepatocytes. *J Clin Invest* 1982; **70**: 63–73

82   Sniderman A, Shapiro S, Marpole D, Skinner B, Teng B, Kwiterovich POJ. Association of coronary atherosclerosis with hypobetalipoproteinemia (increased protein but normal cholesterol levels in human plasma low density (beta) lipoproteins). *Proc Natl Acad Sci USA* 1980; **77**: 604–8

83   Brindley DN, Rolland Y. Possible connections between stress, diabetes, obesity, hypertension, and altered metabolism that may result in atherosclerosis. *Clin Sci* 1989; **77**: 453–61

84   Campbell PJ, Carlson MG, Nurjhan N. Fat metabolism in human obesity. *Am J Physiol* 1994; **266**: E600–E605

85   Coppack SW, Evans RD, Fisher RM *et al.* Adipose tissue metabolism in obesity: lipase action in vivo before and after a mixed meal. *Metabolism* 1992; **41**: 264–72

86   Unger RH. Lipotoxicity in the pathogenesis of obesity-dependent NIDDM. Genetic and clinical implications. *Diabetes* 1995; **44**: 863–70

87   Svedberg J, Bjorntorp P, Smith U, Lonnroth P. Free fatty acid inhibition of insulin binding, degradation and action in isolated rat hepatocytes. *Diabetes* 1990; **39**: 570–4

88   Reaven GM. The fourth musketeer — from Alexander Dumas to Claude Bernard. *Diabetologia* 1995; **38**: 3–13

89   Reynisdottir S, Langin D, Carlstrom K, Holm C, Rossner S, Arner P. Effects of weight reduction on the regulation of lipolysis in adipocytes of women with upper-body obesity. *Clin Sci* 1995; **89**: 421–9

90   Kertzman H, Livshits G, Green MS. Ethnic differences in indices of body mass and body fat distribution. *Int J Obes* 1994; **18**: 69–77

91   Swinburn BA, Craig PL, Daniel R, Dent DPD, Strauss BJD. Body composition differences between Polynesians and Caucasians assessed by bioelectrical impedance. *Int J Obes* 1996; **20**: 889–94

92   McKeigue PM, Shah B, Marmot MG. Relation of central obesity and insulin resistance with high diabetes prevalence and cardiovascular risk in South Asians. *Lancet* 1991; **337**: 382–6

93   McKeigue PM, Pierpoint T, Ferrie JE, Marmot MG. Relationship of glucose intolerance and hyperinsulinaemia to body fat pattern in south Asians and Europeans. *Diabetologia* 1992; **35**: 785–91

94   Chaturvedi N, McKeigue PM, Marmot MG. Relationship of glucose intolerance to coronary risk in Afro-Caribbeans compared with Europeans. *Diabetologia* 1994; **37**: 765–72

95   Dowling HJ, Fried SK, Pi-Sunyer FX. Insulin resistance in adipocytes of obese women; effects of body fat distribution and race. *Metabolism* 1995; **44**: 987–95

Obesity and female reproductive function

R Pettigrew and **D Hamilton-Fairley**

Department of Obstetrics and Gynaecology, St Thomas' Hospital, London, UK

Obesity has consistently been demonstrated to have a detrimental effect upon the female reproductive system. This review explores the common association of obesity with polycystic ovary syndrome (PCOS), the effect of obesity on the clinical and endocrinological parameters, and the role of insulin resistance in the expression of this disorder. An improvement in menstrual function, a decrease in the clinical androgenic profile, and significant increase in spontaneous pregnancy rates have been reported following weight loss. Obesity is associated with poor pregnancy outcome and miscarriage in both women with PCOS, and in those with normal ovarian morphology. The optimal weight gain during pregnancy remains controversial, but obesity is a risk factor for both maternal and fetal complications, and dietary advice should be offered on an individual basis according to the pre-pregnancy BMI. Weight gain at the time of menopause is common, and dietary advice is paramount as obesity is an independent risk factor for thrombosis, coronary heart disease (CHD), and breast and endometrial cancer. Effective nutritional counselling should be offered at all stages of the female reproductive lifecycle.

Obesity is an increasingly common health problem which is an important risk factor in obstetrics and gynaecology, and has been found to affect female reproductive function in several respects. Complications are more prevalent during pregnancy and childbirth, and menstrual disturbance and infertility are frequent consequences of female obesity.

One of the most common gynaecological disorders associated with obesity is polycystic ovary syndrome (PCOS). Insulin resistance is thought to play a central role in the expression of this syndrome, and the relationship between PCOS, obesity and insulin will be discussed in this review. Weight reduction in these women has been shown to improve menstrual function and reduce hyperinsulinaemia, hyperandrogenaemia and peripheral insulin resistance. Women with normal ovarian morphology also are affected adversely by obesity throughout their reproductive life, and this will also be discussed.

There has been much interest and controversy surrounding the ideal weight gain for pregnant women, and the effects of excess weight upon pregnancy outcome in terms of both maternal and fetal morbidity and mortality. The recommendations concerning gestational weight gain and the adverse outcomes associated with obesity in pregnancy are reviewed

Correspondence to:
Miss D Hamilton-Fairley,
Department of Obstetrics
and Gynaecology,
St Thomas' Hospital,
Lambeth Palace Road,
London SE1 7EH, UK

in this chapter. Obesity has consistently been found to have a detrimental effect upon reproductive endocrine function, and weight loss should be encouraged pre-conceptually with nutritional advice being offered during pregnancy.

Polycystic ovary syndrome (PCOS)

Polycystic ovary (PCO) syndrome was initially described by Stein and Leventhal in 1935 as a syndrome of obesity, hirsuitism, anovulation and infertility, associated with enlarged and polycystic ovaries[1]. This is a common heterogeneous disorder; Polson et al. reported the prevalence of PCO morphology in 23% of a large group of asymptomatic women volunteers of reproductive age[2]. There still exists much controversy surrounding the diagnosis, pathophysiology and aetiology of this disorder, as a broad spectrum of symptoms is encompassed by this diagnosis[3].

PCOS may be an incidental finding on a routine ultrasound scan in a woman of normal weight with regular menstrual cycles who does not exhibit signs of hyperandrogenism or, conversely, these women may present with a classical appearance of hirsuitism, obesity and oligo or amenorrhoea. The principal abnormality in women with PCOS is one of anovulation manifested by oligomenorrhoea or secondary amenorrhoea. The diagnostic criteria which are generally agreed upon are based upon the morphological appearance of the ovaries on ultrasound scan, which appears to be a more sensitive marker for PCOS compared with the classical endocrinological features. Accepted criteria describe ovarian morphology with more than 10 peripheral cysts in a single plane, sized between 2–8 mm, arranged in an echodense stroma[4]. This sonographic appearance of PCO may occur together, or in isolation with a biochemical imbalance, which classically involves metabolic and hormonal changes. Concentrations of luteinizing hormone (LH) are elevated in 45–75% of cases in a reported series, and a raised testosterone is seen in 80% of patients[5]; these are the usual biochemical indicators of the presence of this syndrome.

The aetiology of polycystic ovaries has long remained elusive, and the pathophysiology of PCOS is still uncertain. There is increasing evidence that the primary abnormality is excessive ovarian androgen production. It is a minority of women with PCOS who are obese, studies suggesting 35–50%[6,21], but obesity has consistently been shown to increase the prevalence of hirsuitism and anovulation when compared to lean women with PCOS.

Over the last decade, increasing evidence has implicated the role of insulin in the pathophysiology of PCOS. It was first noticed in 1980 by Burghen *et al.* that insulin resistance and PCOS were associated, and there was a correlation between androgen concentration and serum insulin[7]. It was, therefore, hypothesized that obesity and the consequent hyperinsulinaemia might lead to the genesis of PCOS in susceptible individuals[8].

The ovary possesses receptors for both insulin and IGF-1 and there is a cross reactivity between these hormones and their receptors. Thus, hyperinsulinaemia will cause insulin receptors in the ovary to be stimulated directly, and there may be a spill-over effect involving stimulation of IGF-1 receptors. IGF-1 has been shown to potentiate the stimulating effect of follicle stimulating hormone (FSH) on ovarian aromatase activity, on oestradiol and progesterone secretion, and expression of LH receptors[9]. Fasting insulin levels correlate positively with serum IGF-1 and inversely with IGFBP-1 concentrations in lean women with PCOS. IGFBP-1 is a low molecular weight binding protein which is thought to play a central role in regulating the bioavailability of IGF-2, and to a lesser extent IGF-1, and is known to be regulated by insulin. Insulin will cause a decrease in the circulating IGFBP-1 and so increase the potential for IGF-1 to stimulate the ovary. IGF-1 potentiates the action of LH to stimulate the thecal and interstitial components of the ovary[10] and this synergistic effect may lead to an increase in the activity of cytochrome P450c-17alpha hydroxylase, which is an important intermediary in the production of androgens. This LH regulated cytochrome P450 steroidogenic enzyme catalyses the final rate limiting step in testosterone and androstenedione biosynthesis, which is then used as a substrate by the ovarian granulosa cells to convert androgenic precursors to oestrogen. Sharp *et al*[11]. demonstrated that *in vivo*, the major effect of insulin on androgen secretion was mediated by changes in sex hormone binding globulin (SHBG). Insulin levels in a study by Hamilton-Fairley *et al.* were not significantly raised in the PCOS group as a whole, but were elevated in anovulatory compared with ovulatory women[12], despite having similar androgen levels; this may indicate that it is insulin resistance in the ovary that contributes to the mechanism of anovulation, and that insulin is not directly involved in the increased androgen production in these women. Insler's group found that serum IGFBP-1 concentration was inversely correlated to insulin concentration and was significantly lower in obese PCOS than in non obese[13]. They also showed SHBG levels to be significantly lower in obese women, compared to non obese patients. It may thus be postulated that in obese women, hyperinsulinaemia is a secondary disorder, resulting in a decrease in SHBG and IGFBP-1 levels, creating an increase in free androgens, which are in turn converted to

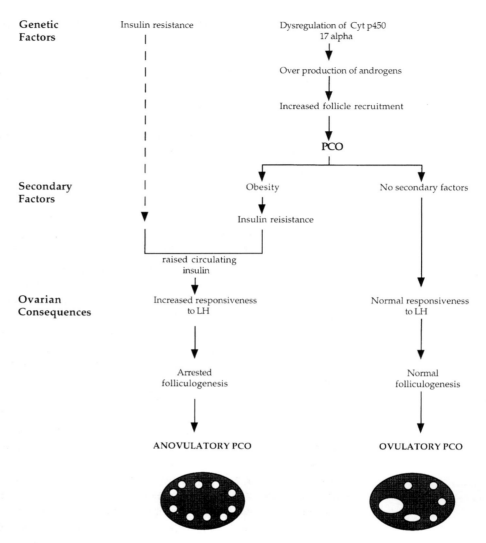

Fig. 1 Diagram illustrating a hypothesis for the pathogenesis of anovulation in PCOS.

oestrone due to the excessive adipose tissue. Figure 1 illustrates a hypothesis for the underlying biochemical abnormality.

Two important factors account for the prevalence of menstrual abnormalities in obese women with PCOS. Firstly, obese women produce more oestrogen by extraglandular conversion of androgens than do non obese subjects and, therefore, have a greater excess of circulating oestrone over oestradiol concentrations than lean women; a positive correlation of the oestradiol/oestrone ratio with BMI has been confirmed by Kiddy *et al*[14]. Secondly, as concentrations of SHBG are much lower in obese women, there is an increased free biologically active fraction of oestradiol in this group of women. Dysfunctional uterine bleeding will often improve after weight loss and up to 80% improvement in menstrual function has been reported following weight loss[15].

Kiddy and colleagues observed a marked improvement in the clinical and endocrinological profile of obese women with PCOS following a long term, low calorie diet (less than 1000 kcal per day over a period of 6–7 months)[16]. This improvement occurred in those women who lost more than 5% of their initial body weight, with an improvement in reproductive function (demonstrated by a 70% spontaneous conception rate) in previously subfertile women who lost weight. Menstrual regularity was also improved and hirsuitism was reduced by 40% in the women in this group. There was no significant change in gonadotrophin concentrations, or total serum testosterone levels, but a marked increase in concentrations of SHBG with a reciprocal change in free testosterone levels. These changes in the weight loss group were accompanied by reduced fasting serum insulin levels, and a decreased response to an oral loading dose of glucose. There is now evidence to suggest that insulin inhibits hepatic secretion of SHBG both *in vivo*[17] and *in vitro*[18]. There were no significant changes in either clinical or endocrine indices in the group who lost less than 5% of their pretreatment weight. The hypothesis suggested is that a reduction in insulin concentrations either directly or indirectly affects ovarian function. These results emphasize the endocrine impact of obesity and body fat distribution. Balen *et al.* also confirmed a positive correlation between body mass index (BMI) with an increased rate of hirsuitism, cycle disturbance, infertility and raised serum testosterone concentrations[19]. Again, therapeutic weight loss was encouraged, and was found to improve the symptoms and endocrine profile of women with PCOS.

Although routine measurement of serum insulin concentration was not recommended, Conway *et al.* reported an 11% prevalence of diabetes in obese PCO patients, which underlines the importance of assessing glucose tolerance in these women[20]. Women who are overweight should be encouraged to lose weight, and can then expect to experience an improvement in the symptoms of menstrual disturbance, infertility and hyperandrogenism. The effects of BMI, however, are part of a spectrum, and the amount of weight loss should not be based on an all or nothing effect with a fixed BMI as an end point, since improvement may occur after a relatively small weight loss.

Hamilton-Fairley *et al.* studied the impact of body weight upon anovulatory women who were undergoing ovulation induction with low dose gonadotrophin therapy, to assess the influence of those women who were moderately overweight upon fecundity and miscarriage rates. Women with marked overweight (BMI more than 28) were excluded from this trial. The conception rate was found to be similar in both groups, but the risk of miscarriage was found to rise with increasing BMI[21]. Overweight women were found to be more likely to receive gonadotrophin therapy, as they were less likely to respond to clomiphene ovulation induction than their lean counterparts[22]. This study further found that overweight women undergoing this treatment required significantly higher doses of gonadotrophins than lean women in order to achieve satisfactory ovarian stimulation. It was apparent that overweight women were relatively resistant to the action of endogenous gonadotrophin, as the levels of mid follicular FSH were appropriate for the higher dose received by the overweight group. Although the conception rate did not appear to be affected between the lean and overweight groups, there was a significant increase in the rate of miscarriage, and appeared to be independent of raised LH concentrations as serum LH levels were similar in both groups. The prevalence of early pregnancy loss in a population of women with PCOS was significantly greater in the overweight group (47%) compared with 27% in the lean group.

The distribution of fat is also important. Pasquali published a report upon the effect of fat distribution on the clinical, hormonal and metabolic features of women with PCOS[23]. After adjustment for BMI and age, the waist to hip ratio (WHR) was found to be positively correlated with an increased LH, androstenedione and oestrone concentrations, as well as higher levels of fasting and glucose stimulated insulin, higher levels of triglycerides, elevated serum very low density lipoprotein (VLDL) and apolipoprotein B, and lower levels of high density lipoprotein (HDL) cholesterol. These results are perhaps not surprising, as it has been previously reported that this android distribution of fat is associated with atherogenesis and poor metabolic parameters. Android obesity is the result of fat deposited in the abdominal wall and visceral mesenteric locations. This fat is more sensitive to catecholamines and less sensitive to insulin, which renders it metabolically more active, with a resulting association of hyperinsulin-aemia and cardiovascular risk factors.

It would appear that obesity is both a result of, and a contributing factor to, the endocrine imbalance in PCOS and these patients will be caught in a vicious circle of increasing hyperandrogenism. Improving matters using dietary restriction requires low carbohydrate diets, and thus provides an endocrine basis for a dietary approach to treatment. The role of insulin in the pathogenesis of PCOS may suggest a future pharmacological treatment in PCOS. As there is no change in ovarian morphology following weight loss, this would suggest, however, that obesity contributes to the clinical and biochemical abnormalities in PCOS, but is not the underlying cause of the disorder. The persistent state of hyperinsulinaemia associated with obesity causes hyperandrogenism, which may also be associated with menstrual irregularities and anovulatory infertility. It is obvious that, in the absence of ovulation, women will fail to become pregnant. The importance of weight loss for those obese women with PCOS must be emphasised, as this may restore ovulation and improve fertility.

Fertility and obesity

Obesity is common among multiparous women but this would suggest that weight gain is the result of many pregnancies, rather than it being a favourable factor for conception. The impact of obesity upon the endocrinological profile has already been discussed, particularly in reference to the relationship of obesity and polycystic ovaries.

There are no data available for fertility rates in obese women who do not have PCOS, but there is evidence for an increased risk of miscarriage. Hamilton-Fairley et al.[21] studied the risk of miscarriage and associated BMI and miscarriage rate in 13,128 primiparous women in the North West Thames region (1992). These data included women with normal ovarian morphology and women with PCOS. Of 9239 women with a BMI of 19–24.9, 11% miscarried. In the moderately overweight group (BMI of 25–27.9), 14% went on to miscarry, which when adjusted for maternal age, represents an odds ratio of 1.26. In the overweight and obese group (BMI greater than 28), 15% of these women miscarried, (the adjusted odds ratio for this group being 1.37). These data confirm that increasing obesity significantly reduces the chances of a successful pregnancy.

The distribution of fat seems to be important in the general population. To assess the effects of this variable upon female fecundity, a prospective cohort study was performed using women attending a fertility clinic requiring donor insemination. The WHR, BMI, age and conception rates were recorded. It was found that the percentage of women who became pregnant fell from 63% to 32% with increasing WHR. Cumulative pregnancy rates for women with WHRs less than 0.8 (gynaecoid obesity) were significantly higher than for women with ratios more than 0.8 (android or central obesity). Both underweight and overweight women had a lower chance of becoming pregnant than women with normal weight, although this effect was greater for obese women than lean women[24]. One hypothesis suggested that an increase in the androgenic microenvironment of the follicle could decrease oocyte quality. Weight loss has been shown to restore cycle regularity, and sex hormone concentrations, which does indicate that it is the obesity which exacerbates reproductive problems.

To assess the effect of morbid obesity on fertility, Bilenka *et al.* studied a group of massively obese women who were undergoing bariatric surgery using vertical banded gastroplasty[25]. The report studied 9 women and their pregnancies before and after treatment and their subsequent weight loss. Of 18 pregnancies prior to the operation, 6 ended in miscarriage. Of the 13 pregnancies following weight loss, only one miscarried. Of this group, the conceptions were all spontaneous, whereas previously, 5 out of 6 attempting to conceive required ovulation induction. Although the numbers were small, this paper demonstrates the importance of excessive weight upon conception rates and the rate of miscarriage.

The relationship between obesity and fertility, and the impact of body fat distribution on miscarriage rates appears to warrant pre-conceptual advice concerning weight loss. Although weight loss is not recommended while pregnant, the presence of obesity, and the related hyperinsulinaemia is thought to be responsible for early pregnancy loss.

Weight gain and pregnancy

Obesity is a common nutritional problem, and many recent studies have assessed the pregnancy course and outcome in association with maternal obesity. However, there remains a lack of consensus on appropriate weight gain in obese pregnant women. This was evident in the 1990 Institute of Medicine report[26], which recommended a minimum weight gain of at least 7 kg (15 lb) for obese women, but due to lack of clear data, was unable to specify an upper limit of weight gain.

Weight gain in pregnancy reflects both fat deposition, a physiological adaptation, and water, due to expansion of the plasma volume and total body water, as well as increases in the size of the uterus and breasts. If weight gain is excessive, the maternal fat stores may not be expended during the pregnancy, and will thus be retained in the postpartum period.

As there is no accepted defining value for obesity in pregnancy, the prevalence is unreported. However, obesity has been reported as increasing in women of reproductive age. A true assessment of the magnitude of this problem is important, and its subsequent effect upon weight gain in the fetus, and maternal and neonatal morbidity and mortality. The BMI is the generally accepted quantifying term for obesity and an important initial assessment of any pregnant woman should involve a calculation of the BMI. Routine measurement of maternal weight gain has been an integral part of prenatal care for many years, but the amount of gain considered desirable has varied over the years. Prospective trials evaluating BMI and correlating this with pregnancy outcome have yet to be performed. The relationship between maternal weight gain and fetal growth is not clear and the range of weight gain which is acceptable to reduce the risk of delivering either macrosomic or small for gestational age babies is still controversial. High and low weight gain in women of ideal weight have been associated with increased frequency of perinatal death[27] and preterm delivery has been associated with low weight gains, particularly in the third trimester. Publications in 1989 concerning weight gain in pregnancy noted that low birth weight was 2.3 times more likely and fetal death was 1.5 times more likely in women who gained less than 20 lb (9 kg) during pregnancy, when compared with those who gained more than 20 lb. It was assumed that there was a direct correlation between the amount of weight gained in pregnancy and the pregnancy outcome in terms of low birth weight babies and infant mortality. Following this report, recommendations of increased weight gain during pregnancy were instituted.

The distribution and range of maternal gain is more variable in obese women, and some studies have reported that women who are obese when pregnancy begins, gain less weight on average than those who are not obese. The relationship concerning obese pregnant women, weight gain and birthweight is uncertain, although it would appear that obese women are at higher risk of both maternal and fetal complications.

Current recommendations from the Institute of Medicine (IOM) suggest a minimum gain of 15 lb (6.8 kg) in obese women, commencing just prior to pregnancy, until delivery at term, with no upper limit specified. However, the pattern of weight gain remains unquantified. Based on the limited literature available, the IOM committee recommended a weekly maternal weight gain of approximately 1 lb (0.45 kg) per week during the second and third trimesters for women of normal pre-pregnancy BMI. Just over 1 lb per week weight gain is recommended for underweight women, and just under for obese gravidas. Because pre-pregnancy weight and body size has been shown to modify the relationship between gestational weight gain and birth weight, separate recommendations are made for under weight, normal weight, over-weight and obese women[28]. Many studies have suggested that the effect of a given weight gain on fetal growth is greatest in thin women and least in overweight women[29,30].

Low maternal weight gain is undesirable due to its association with very low birth weight babies; conversely, high maternal weight gain may be complicated by the difficulties in delivering large infants secondary to clinically overt or subclinical gestational diabetes. Complications arising in pregnancy are often exaggerated in obese mothers. However, it is also true that obese mothers are generally older than their lean counterparts, and, therefore, maternal age may be a confounding factor for the development of medical disorders. Most studies have demonstrated that maternal obesity is an independent factor for the development of diabetes and hypertension. Diabetes is associated with a hyperinsulinaemic state, hyperglycaemia and insulin resistance, which are all conditions which are common in both advancing gestation, and obesity. Gestational diabetes is seen more frequently among obese pregnant women[31] and can also be attributed to insulin resistance. Although gestational diabetes usually resolves shortly following delivery, there remains an increased risk of the mother developing diabetes in later life.

Chronic hypertension is another medical condition which may arise in obese gravidas. Gross *et al.* reported 7% in obese women (compared to 1.5% of lean women) having chronic hypertension[32]. A reported 17% of obese gravidas compared with lean women were noted to develop pre-eclampsia, although there was no significant increase in eclampsia.

Several studies have assessed the intrapartum risk involved for obese women and have shown increased risks associated with high pre-pregnancy BMI and large weight gain during pregnancy. In 1992, Johnson *et al.*[33] performed a longitudinal retrospective study observing 7407 term pregnancies delivered over a 2 year period. 3191 cases were suitable for analysis after elimination for fetal abnormalities, selected medical or surgical complications, and those with no antenatal care or incomplete records. Pregnancy outcome was evaluated in regard to BMI categories recommended by the National Academy of Sciences, that is low (<19.8) medium ($19.8–26$) high ($27–29$) and obese (>29). Increased maternal pre-pregnancy BMI and increased maternal gestational weight gain were both associated with an increased risk of macrosomia ($P<0.0001$)[33]. This study also found that dysfunctional labour was statistically more likely ($P<0.0001$) as was postdatism, meconium staining and unscheduled Caesarean sections. Not surprisingly, low birthweight babies were statistically less frequent. There were significant trends in both weight gain and BMI for the risk of labour abnormalities, even after adjusting for multiple confounding factors. Labour abnormality was cited as the most frequent indication for unscheduled Caesarean section. There was also an increased incidence of oxytocin induction, with a 2-fold increase in the odds ratio for induction in the highest body mass index quartile and a 1.5-fold increase in the highest weight gain category. High pre-pregnancy weight or excessive weight gain has been shown in this and other studies to lead to obstetric complications and, although the incidence of low birth weight babies may be decreased with an adequate increase in weight in leaner women, this principle does not necessarily translate to those women who are obese preconceptually. Therefore, weight gain has to be individualised, and these data indicate that as the pre-pregnancy weight is increased, the recommended gestational weight gain should be decreased.

Serious medical obstetric complications more likely to arise in obese women include hypertension, cardiomyopathy, acute fatty liver of pregnancy (AFLP) and cholestasis in pregnancy, and should be considered during antenatal care. Women who are lean should be treated as a different population, requiring very different nutritional advice to those women who are obese.

Prenatal diagnosis is made more difficult in those women who are grossly obese. Wolfe *et al.* studied the effect of increasing maternal size on ultrasonographic visualisation of fetal anatomy, and found that visualisation of fetal organs was significantly decreased in the obese group. Thus important fetal abnormalities may fail to be detected antenatally.The level of obesity at which visualisation was affected substantially[34,35], was marked, namely a BMI of 36.2.

The obese patient is also at risk for morbidity arising from operative delivery. There is an increased risk of wound infection, urinary tract infection, blood loss, and thromboembolic complications. Should operative delivery be necessary, regional anaesthetic blocks are the anaesthetic of choice due to compromised respiratory function in the obese gravid; this may, however, be technically difficult in an obese patient. If an emergency delivery is necessary, then rapid sequence induction is a technique which is common in obstetric anaesthesia and helps prevent the aspiration of gastric contents.

Postpartum weight retention is another important issue which is related to weight gain in pregnancy. O'Scholl found that women who had a normal pre-pregnancy BMI, and who gained weight at an excessive and essentially unlimited rate, did not greatly enhance fetal growth, but were more likely to develop postpartum obesity[36]. Advancing age and lifestyle changes may be confounding factors, but beginning a subsequent pregnancy with extra weight leads to an increase risk of gestational diabetes, hypertension and the complications in labour which have already been discussed. There is little information available concerning postpartum loss of weight, but the strongest factor contributing to postpartum weight changes is prenatal weight gain. Clinical recommendations from the IOM report suggest that women should generally lose 0.45–0.9 kg per month during the first 6 months postpartum, although there is much variability. Women who are breast feeding need to be encouraged to consume at least 1800 kcal per day, and any intake below this is not recommended. Obese women, however, can aim to lose up to 2 kg per month without jeopardising their milk quality, although losing weight within the first few weeks postpartum is generally not recommended, as this is the point at which milk supply is being established[36].

Obesity is a severe health hazard, and adequate nutritional advice should be given to all pregnant women. Obesity is associated with an increased risk of miscarriage, but those fortunate enough to have an ongoing pregnancy need particular attention, and regular antenatal screening for glucose intolerance, hypertension, macrosomia and excessive weight gain should be routine. The mother can then be counselled appropriately throughout her pregnancy. Nutritional advice should be altered according to the individual depending upon the pre-pregnancy weight, and weight gain recommendations in obese women should vary from that advice given to lean pregnant women. Weight loss postpartum must also be encouraged, particularly in those women retaining weight, and they need to be assisted in attaining their ideal weight[37].

Hormone replacement therapy (HRT) and obesity

The menopause is defined as one year following the last menstrual period; the median age of menopause in most developed societies is around 50 years. The essential feature of the menopause is the failure of ovarian follicular development. A finite number of oocytes are laid down in fetal life (about 7 million) with approximately 450,000 oocytes being available by puberty. It is thought that once this number has reached critically low levels, then irreversible ovarian failure occurs. In premenopausal women, the follicle is responsible for more than 90% of oestradiol produced, and when folliculogenesis ceases serum levels of oestradiol decline. Associated with this is an increase in FSH and LH, thus giving the characteristic biochemical picture of hypergonadotrophic hypogonadism. The postmenopausal ovary does secrete some oestradiol, but most is produced by peripheral conversion from androgens. Androstenedione is the most important androgen used for the production of oestrogens. It is a C19 steroid which exhibits little androgenic activity, and is converted in the liver and adipose tissue to oestrone. The production of adrenal androgens is related to body weight and it is, therefore, likely that the higher amount of oestrogen produced in obese women is due to a higher production of androgen precursor, as well as its higher rate of aromatisation in adipose tissue. Menopause has been associated with increases in upper body (android) fat distribution. Oestrogen is thought to promote a gynaecoid fat distribution, which carries less risk for diabetes, and cardiovascular risk factors than android fat deposition.

A low oestrogen status causes several symptoms to a woman who is peri or postmenopausal. The vasomotor flush is the hallmark feature.

Oestrogen deficiency causes atrophic changes in the urethra and vagina which may present as dyspareunia, pruritis, vaginitis or urinary frequency and dysuria. Oestrogen deficiency also changes trabecular bone and is thus important in the genesis of osteoporosis. The risk of fracture from osteoporosis is known to be dependant upon bone mass at the time of menopause, and the rate of bone loss following the menopause. In general, bone mass is higher in obese women and in the Afro-Carribean population, and lower in thin, white women who lead sedentary lives. Oestrogen therapy will act prophylactically to prevent osteoporosis or stabilize the process. Epidemiological evidence suggests that oestrogen therapy decreases hip and arm fractures by 50–60%[38]. This reduction is seen primarily in patients who have taken oestrogen for more than 5 years. The annual mortality from hip fractures in women is high and oestrogen replacement will considerably reduce the associated morbidity and mortality rate. A number of studies show that obesity is protective against osteoporosis. Pocock and colleagues demonstrated that the BMI was an important predictor of bone mass in the lumbar spine, distal forearm and femur[39]. This effect is thought to be due both from the mechanical stress which excess body weight places upon the musculoskeletal system, as well as increased postmenopausal oestrogen concentrations. This theory was supported by Krolner, who observed that in patients who had undergone gastric bypass operations, the degree of loss of mineral content in the lumbar spine was closely associated with the degree of weight loss, and hence mechanical stress[40] and was not related to calcium and vitamin D absorption, which would remain unaffected in these patients. The increased synthesis of oestrogen via the conversion of androstenedione into oestrogen in adipocytes is thought to offer an explanation why skeletal regions which are not exposed to any weight related stress also benefit from the protective effect associated with an increased BMI. In a review of lifestyle, obesity, and osteoporosis, Notelovitz reported that untreated menopause, particularly if naturally premature or surgically induced, frequently overrides the protective effect of obesity and following bone density evaluation in their patients, they found that most women required hormone additive therapy[41].

Coronary heart disease (CHD) is now the leading cause of death in women and the risk of this disease markedly rises following the loss of ovarian function. During the reproductive years, women are protected from coronary heart disease, presumably by the raised serum levels of high density lipoprotein (HDL). Oestrogen replacement therapy increase the HDLs and reduces LDL (low density lipoprotein) and cholesterol levels[42]. HRT has been found to reduce the incidence of CHD in postmenopausal women by up to 50%. Obesity is a risk factor for the development of CHD and, therefore, an additional risk would be a prolonged low oestrogen state. HRT causes changes in lipids and lipoprotein profiles[42]. The effects of gonadal steroid hormones have important influences upon the cardiovascular system, and these non lipid effects may contribute to the pathogenesis of CHD. These include direct arterial effects as well as the metabolic consequences of insulin resistance and hyperinsulinaemia[43]. Oestradiol reverses the effects of menopause on glucose and insulin metabolism, causing insulin resistance to be decreased. Androgenic progestagens may oppose this potentially beneficial effect on insulin resistance. HRT also reverses the increased central fat distribution, which is associated with atherogenic biochemical parameters.

Breast cancer and endometrial cancer are increased by long term oestrogen replacement therapy. The incidence of endometrial carcinoma is increased in women who are obese, nulliparous and infertile. Obese women already have a substantially increased risk of developing endometrial cancer, varying from 3 times normal when 9.5–22.5 kg overweight, to 10 times when the excess of weight is greater than 22.5 kg[44]. A close correlation has also been shown between daily dietary fat consumption and the development of endometrial cancer[45]. The increased peripheral conversion of androgens to oestrogens, and the resultant effect of the unopposed oestrogen upon the endometrium is thought to be responsible. Women who use unopposed oestrogens have a dose dependent risk of developing endometrial cancer, but current knowledge assumes that mortality can be reduced by an increase in clinical surveillance. Women who take progestogens with the oestrogen are protected from any increased risk of developing endometrial cancer. Risks for postmenopausal breast cancer have been identified as obesity, late age at menopause, a family history of breast disease and an early age at menarche. The association between HRT and breast cancer is weak and controversial. Thrombosis is a further reported risk factor in HRT use, but current evidence would suggest that the arterial risks associated with obesity are not significantly worsened by the administration of HRT. In 1988, Henderson et al.[46] reviewed literature on mortality from osteoporotic hip fractures, endometrial cancer, breast cancer and ischaemic heart disease in women aged 65–74 years and calculated the hypothetical risk from postmenopausal oestrogen use in each of these diseases. The total mortality from coronary heart disease and osteoporotic hip fractures is many times greater than from breast cancer and, therefore, on balance, the beneficial effects of therapy appear to outweigh the small increased risk of breast cancer. The addition of progestagens considerably decreases the risk of endometrial cancer.

The relationship between obesity and weight gain with postmenopausal hormone replacement therapy remains uncertain. While weight gain is common at the time of the menopause, it has also been suggested that oestrogen replacement is directly associated with an increased prevalence of obesity. There have been several studies upon the effect of HRT on fat distribution, which have yielded contradictory results. Several of these studies have found HRT use associated with lower WHRs, although other centres have reported that, after correcting for age and degree of obesity, this correlation disappears. In a randomised prospective trial using a cross sectional cohort over a 15 year period by Kritz-Silverstein *et al.*, it appeared that women using intermittent or continuous hormone replacement therapy, had significantly lower mean BMIs at baseline than women who never used HRT. After adjustment for potentially confounding covariates, there were no significant differences between oestrogen users, and those not on oestrogen replacement in BMI at follow up, change in weight or BMI between baseline and follow up, or WHR or fat mass at follow up, thereby suggesting no association between HRT and weight gain and the central obesity distribution of fat that is common in postmenopausal women[47]. Weight gain seen around the time of the menopause is multifactorial and varies substantially within ethnic and socioeconomic groups and may be more related to age and lifestyle changes, rather than to the effect of postmenopausal oestrogen therapy.

Obesity at the time of the menopause is a common occurrence and justifies dietary advice and therapeutic action. Central obesity increases the risk from CHD, and the postmenopausal state is associated with more atherogenic lipid profiles. Treatment with oral exogenous oestrogens induces favourable effects on lipids and lipoproteins, and epidemiological evidence has established that the risk of cardiovascular mortality is reduced by 40–60% in women receiving HRT. Although obesity does confer a protective effect upon bone loss in menopausal women, evidence would again suggest that mortality from osteoporotic fractures is considerably reduced in women using HRT. The controversial link between exogenous oestrogen use in peri and postmenopausal women and breast cancer has not been established, and with increased surveillance for endometrial carcinoma, the relative benefits conferred upon both obese and non obese postmenopausal women would appear to outweigh the detrimental effects of HRT.

Conclusions

The implications and consequences of obesity are far reaching and obese women trying to become pregnant, or those who have already conceived, will require advice on the effects of their body mass upon conception rates, and the risks and complications associated with pregnancy and childbirth. Those women with PCOS must be strongly encouraged to lose weight in order to improve their menstrual function and androgenic profile. Hirsuitism and subfertility may be effectively treated with a simple weight loss regimen, and may result in spontaneous ovulation, thereby avoiding the need for ovulation induction using pharmacological intervention. Should a pregnancy be achieved, both women with PCOS **and** those with normal ovarian morphology who are obese are at a significantly greater risk of miscarriage, and nutritional advice and counselling should be offered at the earliest opportunity. Regular antenatal screening should be offered to monitor blood pressure, maternal weight gain, glucose tolerance, and a sonographic assessment of fetal growth to exclude macrosomia. These women should be advised of potential complications that may arise during the delivery and while weight loss is not recommended in pregnancy, weight gain should be restricted and monitored carefully. HRT is generally agreed to be beneficial for postmenopausal women and, although body mass and obesity confer a degree of protection against osteoporosis, studies have demonstrated that exogenous hormone replacement is still important to prevent CHD and osteoporotic changes, and the benefits of this therapy would appear to outweigh the disadvantages.

References

1   Stein IF, Leventhal ML. Amenorrhoea associated with bilateral polycystic ovaries. *Ann J Obstet Gynecol* 1935; **29**: 181–91

2   Polson DW, Adams J, Wadsworth J, Franks S. Polycystic ovaries—a common finding in normal women. *Lancet* 1988; i: 870–2

3   Franks S. Polycystic ovary syndrome—a changing perspective. *Clin Endocrinol* 1989; **31**: 87–120

4   Adams J, Franks S, Polson DW *et al*. Multifollicular ovaries: clinical and endocrine features and response to pulsatile gonadotrophin releasing hormone. *Lancet* 1985; ii: 1375–8

5   Robinson S, Kiddy D, Gelding S *et al*. Decreased insulin sensitivity in women with polycystic ovaries is related to menstrual disturbance. *Clin Endocrinol* 1993: **39**; 368–71

6   Singh KB, Mahajan DK, Wortsman J. Effect of obesity on the hormonal characteristics of the polycystic ovary syndrome. *J Reprod Med* 1990: **39**: 805–8

7   Burghen GA, Givens JR, Kitabci AE. Correlation of hyperandrogenism with hyperinsulinaemia in polycystic ovarian disease. *J Clin Endocrinol Metab* 1980; **50**: 113–5

8   Nestler JE, Clore JN, Blackard WG. The central role of obesity (hyperinsulinaemia) in the pathogenesis of the polycystic ovary syndrome. *Am J Obstet Gynecol* 1989; **161**: 1095–7

9   Adashi EY, Resnick CE, Hernandez ER *et al*. Insulin-like growth factor-1 as an amplifier of follicle stimulating hormone action: studies on mechanisms and sites of action in cultured rat granulosa cells. *Endocrinology* 1988; **122**; 1583–91

10 Cara JF, Fan J, Azzraello J, Rosenfield RL. Insulin like growth factor 1 enhances luteinizing hormone binding to rat ovarian theca-interstsitial cells. *J Clin Invest* 1990; **86**: 560–5

11 Sharp PS, Kiddy DS, Reed MJ, Anyaoku V, Johnstone DG, Franks S. Correlation of plasma insulin and insulin like growth factor-1 with indices of androgen transport and metabolism in women with polycystic ovary syndrome. *Clin Endocrinol* 1991; **35**: 253–7

12 Hamilton-Fairley D, Kiddy D, Anyaoku V, Koistinen R, Seppala M, Franks S. Response of sex hormone binding globulin and insulin-like growth factor binding protein-1 to an oral glucose

tolerance test in obese women with polcystic ovary syndrome before and after calorie restriction. *Clin Endocrinol* 1993: **39**: 363–7

13 Insler V, Shoham Z, Barash A *et al*. Polycystic ovaries in non obese and obese patients: possible pathophysiological mechanisms based on new interpretation of facts and findings. *Hum Reprod* 1993; **8**: 379–84

14 Kiddy DS, Sharp PS, White DM *et al*. Differences in clinical and endocrine features between obese and non obese subjects with polycystic ovary syndrome: an analysis of 263 consecutive cases. *Clin Endocrinol* 1990; **32**: 213–20

15 Hollmann M, Runnebaum B, Gerhard I. Effects of weight loss on the hormonal profile in obese, infertile women. *Hum Reprod* 1996: **11**; 1884–91

16 Kiddy DS, Hamilton-Fairley D, Bush A *et al*. Improvement in endocrine and ovarian function during dietary treatment of obese women with polycystic ovarian syndrome. *Clin Endocrinol* 1992; **36**: 105–11

17 Weaver JU, Holly JMP, Kopelman PG *et al*. Decreased sex hormone binding globulin (SHBG) and insulin like growth factor binding protein-1 (IGFBP-1) in extreme obesity. *Clin Endocrinol* 1990; **33**: 415–22

18 Singh A, Hamilton-Fairley DH, Koistenen R *et al*. Effect of insulin like growth factor type 1 (IGF-1) and insulin on the secretion of sex hormone binding globulin and insulin like growth factor binding protein-1 (IGFBP-1) by human hepatoma cells. *J Endocrinol* 1990; **124**: R1–R3

19 Balen AH, Conway GS, Kaltsas G *et al*. Polycystic ovary syndrome: the spectrum of the disorder in 1741 patients. *Hum Reprod* 1995; **10**: 2107–11

20 Conway GS, Agrawal R, Betteridge DJ, Jacobs HS. Risk factors for coronary artery disease in lean and obese women with the polycystic ovary syndrome. *Clin Endocrinol* 1992; **37**: 119–25

21 Hamilton-Fairley D, Kiddy D, Watson H, Paterson C, Franks S. Association of moderate obesity with a poor pregnancy outcome in women with polycystic ovary syndrome treated with low dose gonadotrophin. *Br J Obstet Gynaecol* 1992; **99**: 128–31

22 Polson DW, Kiddy DS, Mason HD, Franks S. Induction of ovulation with clomiphene citrate in women with polycystic ovary syndrome: the difference between responders and non responders. *Fertil Steril* 1989; **51**: 30–4

23 Pasquali R, Casimirri F, Venturoli S *et al*. Body fat distribution has weight independent effects on clinical and metabolic features of women with polycystic ovary syndrome. *Metabolism* 1994; **43**: 706–13

24 Zaadstra BM, Seidell JC, Van Noord PAH *et al*. Fat and female fecundity: prospective study of effect of body fat distribution on conception rates. *BMJ* 1993; **306**: 484–7

25 Bilenka B, Ben-Shlomo I, Cozacov C, Gold CH, Zohar S. Fertility, miscarriage and pregnancy after vertical banded gastroplasty operation for morbid obesity. *Acta Obstet Gynaecol Scand* 1995; **74**: 42–4

26 Institute of Medicine subcommittee on nutritional status and weight gain during pregnancy. *Nutrition during Pregnancy*. Washington DC: National Academy Press; 1990

27 Naeye RL. Weight gain and the outcome of pregnancy. *Am J Obstet Gynecol* 1979; **135**: 3–9

28 Siega-Riz AM, Adair LS, Hobel CJ. Institute of Medicine maternal weight gain recommendations and pregnancy outcome in a predominantly Hispanic population. *Obstet Gynecol* 1994; **84**: 565–73

29 Abrams B, Laros RK. Prepregnancy weight, weight gain and birth weight. *Am J Obstet Gynecol* 1986; **154**: 504–9

30 Wolfe HM, Zadpr IE, Gross TL, Martier SS, Sokol RJ. The clinical utility of maternal body mass index in pregnancy. *Am J Obstet Gynecol* 1991; **164**: 1307–10

31 Edwards LE, Dickes WF, Alton IR. Pregnancy in the massively obese. Course outcome and obesity prognosis of the infant. *Am J Obstet Gynecol* 1978; **131**: 479–83

32 Gross TL, Sokol RJ, King KC. Obesity in pregnancy: risks and outcome. *Obstet Gynecol* 1980; **56**: 446–50

33 Johnson JWC, Longmate JA, Frentzen B. Excessive maternal weight and pregnancy outcome. *Am J Obstet Gynecol* 1992; **167**: 353–70

34 Wolfe HM, Sokol RJ, Martier SM, Zador IE. Maternal obesity: a potential source of error in sonographic prenatal diagnosis. *Obstet Gynecol* 1990; **76**: 339–42

35 Wolfe HM, Gross TL. Obesity in pregnancy. *Clin Obstet Gynecol* 1994: 37; 596–604

36 O'Scholl T, Hediger ML, Schall JI, Ances IG, Smith WK. Gestational weight gain, pregnancy outcome, and postpartum weight retention. *Am J Obstet Gynecol* 1995; **86**: 423–7

37 Parker JD. Post partum weight change. *Clin Obstet Gynecol* 1994; **37**: 528–37

38 Kiel DP, Felson DT, Anderson JJ, Wilson PWF, Mokowitz MA. Hip fracture and the use of oestrogen in postmenopausal women: the Framingham study. *N Engl J Med* 1987; **317**: 1169

39 Pocock N, Eisman J, Gwinn T *et al*. Muscle strength, physical fitness and weight but not age predict femoral neck bone mass. *J Bone Miner Res* 1989; **4**: 441–8

40 Krolner B, Ranlov PJ, Clemmesen T, Nielson SP. Bone loss after gastroplasty for morbid obesity: side effect or adaptive response to weight loss. *Lancet* 1982; i: 956–7

41 Notelovitz M. Lifestyle, exercise and osteoporosis. In: Drife JO, Studd JW, eds. *HRT and Osteoporosis*. London: Springer, 1990; 323–47

42 Bush TL, Miller VG. Effects of pharmacological agents used during menopause: impact on lipids and lipoproteins. In: Mishell DRJ, ed. *Menopause: Physiology and Pharmacology*. Chicago: Year Book Medical Publishers, 1987: 187–208

43 Stevenson JC, Crook D, Goddsland IF, Collins P, Whitehead MI. Hormone replacement therapy and the cardiovascular system. Non lipid effects. *Drugs* 1994; **47**: 35–41

44 Wynder EL, Escher GC, Mantel N. An epidemiological investigation of cancer of the endometrium. *Cancer* 1966; **19**: 489–520

45 Armstrong B, Doll R. Environmental factors and cancer incidence and mortality in different countries, with special references to dietary practices. *Int J Cancer* 1975; **15**: 617–31

46 Henderson BE, Ross RK, Lobo RA, Pike MC, Mack TM. Re-evaluating the role of progestogen therapy after the menopause. *Fertil Steril* 1988; **49** (**Suppl**): 9S–15S

47 Kritz-Silverstein D, Barrett-Connor E. Long term post menopausal hormone use, obesity, and fat distribution in older women. *JAMA* 1996; **275**: 46–9

Key issues in the prevention of obesity

Timothy P Gill

Post Graduate Nutrition and Dietetic Centre, Rowett Research Institute, Aberdeen, UK

Obesity is a serious, chronic medical condition which is associated with a wide range of debilitating and life-threatening conditions. It imposes huge financial burdens on health care systems and the community at large. Obesity develops over time and once it has done so, is difficult to treat. Therefore, the prevention of weight gain offers the only truly effective means of controlling obesity. Very little research has directly addressed the issue of obesity prevention and previous efforts to prevent obesity amongst individuals, groups or whole communities have had very limited success. However, we have learned sufficient from past preventive activities to realise that the management of obesity will require a comprehensive range of strategies with actions that target those with existing weight problems, those at high risk of developing obesity as well as the community as a whole. The prevention and management of obesity in children should be considered a priority as there is a high risk of persistence into adulthood.

Obesity is a serious medical condition which is associated with a wide range of debilitating, chronic and life-threatening conditions. It imposes huge financial burdens on health care systems and the community at large. The fact that obesity prevalence continues to increase at an alarming rate in almost all regions of the world is, therefore, of major concern. However, despite the potential gains to be achieved from reducing the incidence and prevalence of obesity in a population, surprisingly little attention has so far been given to developing strategies aimed at the prevention of obesity. This chapter examines the key role that prevention should play in the management of obesity and identifies potential prevention strategies and priority areas for action.

The rationale behind obesity prevention

Correspondence to:
Dr Timothy P Gill,
Post Graduate Nutrition
and Dietetic Centre,
Rowett Research Institute,
Greenburn Road,
Bucksburn,
Aberdeen AB21 9SB, UK

The rationale behind obesity prevention is several fold. First, obesity develops over time and, once it has done so, is very difficult to treat. A number of analyses have identified the failure of obesity treatments (with the possible exception of gastric surgery in the seriously obese) to achieve long-term success[1–3]. Second, the health consequences associated with obesity result from the cumulative metabolic and physical stress of excess weight over a long period of time and may not be fully reversible by weight loss[4,5]. Third, the proportion of the population that is either overweight or obese in many developed countries is now so large that there are no longer sufficient health care resources to offer treatment to all[6]. It can be argued, therefore, that the prevention of weight gain (or the reversal of small gains) would be easier, less expensive, and potentially more effective than to treat obesity after it has fully developed.

Is obesity preventable?

The fact that obesity prevalence is rising rapidly and unchecked in almost all areas of the world has led some people to question whether it is possible to prevent excessive gains in body weight over time. However, as mentioned previously, there has so far been little research addressing this question comprehensively. There has only been one controlled intervention study published to date that has been specifically aimed at preventing weight gain in adults. Forster et al.[7] found that after 1 year of a low impact programme (involving four nutrition education sessions, a monthly weight control information newsletter, and an incentive program), those in the treated group had lost about 1 kg in weight, while the weights of those in the control group remained unchanged. Further subgroup analysis showed that the greatest impact was among men, individuals over the age of 50, non-smokers, and those with little prior experience with formal weight loss services. The results of this short-term study are not sufficient to inspire confidence in our ability to prevent obesity.

Indirect evidence from a variety of sources, however, indicates that obesity prevention strategies could indeed prove to be effective in combating the escalating problem of obesity. Given a suitable environment, many people are able to control their weight successfully over long periods of time. This is true both from an individual and from a population perspective. In certain parts of the world such as Japan, for example, the fact that obesity rates are currently low suggests that humans are not biologically destined to become obese. Furthermore, the explosion in rates of obesity has mirrored similar epidemics in non-communicable diseases such as coronary heart disease which are now abating in countries where preventive strategies to deal with these have been adopted. Comprehensive obesity prevention programmes have been introduced very recently in a small number of countries (e.g. Singapore), but not enough time has yet elapsed to be able to evaluate their success. However, the level of obesity in Finnish men from higher education grades has shown a decline since 1985[72].

Perhaps the strongest evidence for the preventability of obesity comes from the successful management of childhood obesity. A number of researchers[8-11] have shown that effective management and support of overweight and obese children can significantly reduce the number of children who carry their weight problem into adulthood. The long term prevention of weight gain in these studies was achieved during the difficult transition periods of childhood and adolescence when weight gain can be a major problem. It is also interesting that in studies where children were treated together with their parents, the children were successful in reducing and maintaining their weight loss whilst over time the adults returned to their pre-study body weight[8].

Obesity prevention strategies

The aims of obesity prevention

The effective control of obesity requires the development of coherent strategies that tackle the main issues relating to the prevention of: (i) the development of overweight in normal weight individuals; (ii) the progression of overweight to obesity in those who are already overweight; (iii) weight regain in those who have been overweight or obese in the past but who have since lost weight; and (iv) further worsening of a condition already established. This involves action at several levels.

Levels of preventive action

The traditional classification of prevention interventions into primary, secondary and tertiary was originally developed to describe actions in relation to acute conditions with an identifiable, unifactoral cause. The objective of primary prevention was seen as decreasing the number of new cases (incidence): secondary prevention was to lower the rate of established cases in the community (prevalence); and tertiary prevention was to stabilise or reduce the amount of disability associated with the disorder. Thus, attention is focused on individual risk factors when applying this system to a multi-factorial condition such as coronary heart disease (CHD). Primary prevention of CHD might involve national programmes to control blood cholesterol levels; secondary prevention may deal with reducing CHD risk in those with existing elevated blood cholesterol levels; and tertiary action would be associated with preventing re-infarction in those who had a previous heart attack. Use of the traditional classification system for obesity prevention strategies, however, results in a great deal of ambiguity and confusion. For example, does primary obesity prevention refer to the prevention of overweight people from becoming obese, or is this secondary prevention. Is tertiary prevention concerned with the prevention of obesity progressing into more severe obesity or rather with the control of co-morbid conditions such as hypertension.

To avoid confusion when discussing strategies for the prevention of chronic, multi-factorial conditions such as obesity, the US Institute of Medicine[12] has proposed an alternative classification system to the traditional one outlined above. The new system separates prevention efforts into three levels: universal or public health measures (directed at everyone in the population); selective (for a subgroup who may have an above average risk of developing obesity); and indicated (targeted at high risk individuals who may have a detectable amount of excess weight which foreshadows obesity (see Fig. 1). In this scheme, prevention is used to describe only those actions that occur before the full development of the condition. Many actions concerned with reducing the disability associated with obesity, previously classified as tertiary prevention, are redefined as maintenance interventions.

Indicated prevention

Indicated prevention deals with individuals who are already overweight or showing biological markers associated with excessive fat stores but who are not yet obese. These are high risk individuals in whom failure to intervene at this stage will result in many becoming obese and suffering the associated ill health consequences in the future.

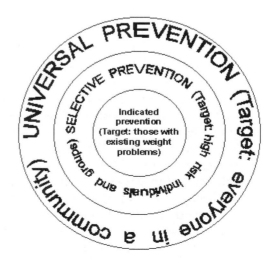

Fig. 1 Levels of prevention measures. This diagram represents the three complementary levels of preventive actions from the very specific indicated prevention approach, to targeted preventive actions and the broader universal or population-wide prevention programmes. Adapted from Institute of Medicine, 1994.

The identification of people who are likely to benefit from indicated prevention programmes should be a component of all clinical assessment protocols in routine health care. Regular determination of body weight and the calculation of body mass index (BMI) identifies patients who have made substantial gains in weight over a short period of time or whose BMI is already at an unhealthy level. In addition, measuring blood pressure and biochemical parameters (such as blood lipids and blood glucose) will indicate when the excessive adiposity is beginning to impact on health.

The recently released Scottish Intercollegiate Guidelines Network (SIGN) report for the management of obesity in Scotland[13] recommends regular screening of body weight and waist measurement. The guidelines suggest that patients should be recruited into indicated preventive programmes through self-referral, practice audit or opportunistic screening. Individuals from families with a history of obesity, or who come from one of the high risk groups or vulnerable periods of life identified in Tables 1 and 2 should be particular targets of these preventive measures. Overweight children ought to be a major focus of such programmes.

Indicated prevention strategies usually involve working with patients on a one-to-one basis or, alternatively, through the establishment of special groups to provide guidance and support. Patients recruited to indicated prevention programmes will already be demonstrating some weight-related problems. Thus, the primary objectives of this preventive strategy are restricted to preventing further weight gain and reducing the number of people who develop obesity-related comorbidities. In particular, indicated prevention aims to prevent overweight children from becoming obese adults.

Selective prevention

Selective prevention measures are aimed at sub-groups of the population who are at a high risk for the development of obesity. High risk sub-groups possess a biological, psychological or socio-cultural factor which has been associated with increased risk for obesity and are identified in Tables 1 and 2. This risk may be acute, as in the case of certain vulnerable life stages, or it may be a life-long concern such as a genetic predisposition to weight gain.

In contrast to the individual patient focus of indicated prevention, selective prevention strategies are directed mostly at groups. These may be initiated through schools, colleges, work sites, community centres and

Table 1 Vulnerable periods of life for the development of future obesity

Vulnerable period	Reason for increased risk
Pre–natal	There is evidence to suggest that fetal nutrition and *in-utero* development has permanent effects on later growth, body shape, fatness and energy regulation[88,99]
Adiposity rebound (5–7 years)	Body mass index begins to increase rapidly after a period of reduced adiposity during pre-school years. Food and activity patterns often change as a result of exposure to new environments and patterns of behaviour conducive to the development of obesity may develop. Early and rapid adiposity rebound indicates increased risk of persistent obesity later in life[89,100]
Adolescence	Period of increased autonomy which is often associated with irregular meals, changed food habits and periods of inactivity during leisure combined with physiological changes which promote increased fat deposition, particularly in females[90,101]
Early adulthood	Early adulthood usually correlates to a period of marked reduction in physical activity. In women this usually occurs between the ages of 15–19 years but in men it may be as late as the early 30s[91]
Pregnancy	Although on average, women gain less than one kilogram after each pregnancy[102], excessive weight gain during pregnancy may result in increased retention of weight after delivery, particularly with early cessation of breastfeeding. This pattern is often repeated after each pregnancy[92]
Menopause	In Western societies, weight generally increases with age but it is not certain why menopausal women are particularly prone to rapid weight gain[93]. The loss of the menstrual cycle does affect food intake and reduce metabolic rate slightly but reduced activity may account for the greatest proportion of this weight gain[103].

Table 2 Identifying groups at high risk of weight gain

High risk groups	Reason for increased risk
Genetically susceptible individuals	There is no longer any doubt that, given the same environment, some individuals are more prone to depositing fat. The basis of these differences in individual susceptibility to obesity is yet to be fully elucidated but is believed to involve a number of physiological processes associated with fat deposition, oxidation and involuntary energy expenditure[94].
Certain ethnic groups	In many countries, certain ethnic groups appear to be especially prone to the development of obesity. This is believed to be the result of a genetic predisposition to obesity which becomes apparent when such groups are exposed to diet and lifestyle patterns conducive to weight gain (e.g. Indian immigrants to the United Kingdom[95]).
Socially or economically disadvantaged	In the United Kingdom and other European countries, there is an inverse association between income and education level and obesity which is most pronounced among women and children. It is argued that cheaper foodstuffs are usually high in fat and energy dense, and those with less financial resources spend more time in sedentary activities such as watching TV[96,98].
Recent successful weight reducers	Successful weight reduction is usually followed by the regain of one–half to one-third of the weight loss over the following year[104]. It is believed that biological and behavioural processes act to drive body weight back to baseline levels[91].
Recent past smokers	Smokers are usually thinner than non–smokers because smoking tends to depress appetite, increase the basal metabolic rate and, after each cigarette, induce a surge in heart and metabolic rate[97]. Mean weight gain attributable to smoking cessation has been found to be on average 2.8 kg in men and 3.8 kg in women but heavy smokers (more than 15 cigarettes per day) and younger people tend to gain much more[100]. However the health benefits of smoking cessation far outweigh the health risks of any subsequent weight gain.
Patients who have been prescribed certain drugs that promote weight gain	A number of classes of drugs are known to promote weight gain mostly through encouraging excessive food intake, often at times of enforced inactivity. Corticosteroids, sulphonylureas, Insulin, β-adrenergic blockers, some steroid contraceptives, goitrogens and other drugs have been associated with weight gain.

shopping outlets as well as primary care settings. Selective prevention is concerned with improving the knowledge and skills of groups of people to allow them to deal more effectively with the factors which put them at a high risk of developing obesity.

Universal or public health prevention

Universal prevention programmes are directed at the population or community as a whole regardless of their current level of risk. Such a mass approach to the control and prevention of lifestyle diseases is not always appropriate and has been criticised for requiring those who may be at low risk to make similar changes to those at high risk[14]. In the prevention of overweight and obesity, however, where the prevalence of the condition is already extremely high and a large proportion of the population is at high risk, universal approaches have the potential to be the most cost effective form of prevention[15].

Universal prevention aims to stabilise the level of obesity in the population, to reduce the incidence of new cases and, eventually, to reduce the prevalence of obesity. However, in line with other public health approaches to disease control, the most important issue in dealing with a problem of extremes in weight is a reduction in the mean weight of the population. The association between the mean level of BMI and the prevalence of obesity is discussed later in the chapter. Other objectives of universal prevention include a reduction in weight-related ill health, improvements in general diet and exercise levels and a reduction in the level of population risk of obesity.

Integrating prevention into management

The reluctance of the medical profession to take up the issue of obesity prevention has been ascribed to: (i) a misunderstanding of the relationship between weight and health; and (ii) a conviction that, given their limited time and health promotion skills, their role is best limited to therapeutic interventions[16].

There has been much controversy over the relationship between body weight and total mortality. Many studies have shown a U or J shaped association between the two, with higher mortality rates at both upper and lower body weights, and where substantial increases in relative risk for mortality do not occur until a BMI around 27–28 kg/m^2 is reached[17–19]. As a result, many health professionals have argued that intervening to control weight gain at levels much below a BMI of 27 kg/m^2 is actually counterproductive to health[20,21]. However, recent re-analyses of these

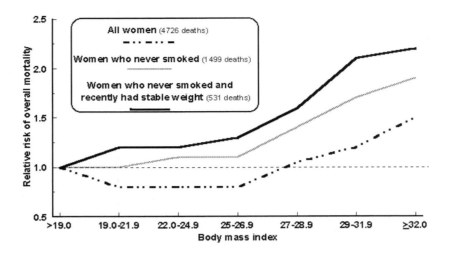

Fig. 2 The relationship between body mass index and relative risk of premature mortality. This figure demonstrates the more linear and continuous relationship between body mass index and premature mortality that emerges when potential confounding factors such as smoking and unintentional weight loss are controlled. It is based on the data presented in Manson et al [24]. Although this study was only conducted in middle-aged women, it was well controlled and had a large sample size. The findings are consistent with other information on the relationship between BMI and morbidity and mortality. [Adapted from Manson et al. 1995[24].]

studies have revealed that they contained a number of biases including cigarette smoking, weight loss associated with illness and lack of age standardisation which lead to a systematic under-estimation of the impact of obesity on premature mortality[22,23]. In addition, many of these studies inappropriately controlled for hypertension and other conditions on the assumption that these were confounding factors when they are, to a large degree, the effects of obesity.

More recent studies[24,25] that have appropriately controlled for confounding factors have found an almost linear, continuous association between BMI and mortality with no specific threshold (see Fig. 2). This is not surprising given the largely linear relationship between body weight and conditions such as coronary heart disease, hypertension and non-insulin dependent diabetes as BMI increases from 20 kg/m² to 30 kg/m² [26–28]. An analysis of numerous studies of obesity and mortality risk by the American Institute of Nutrition[29], concluded that the lowest mortality risk is associated with BMIs of 18–25 kg/m². The rise in mortality with increasing relative weight is steeper in men and women under 50 years of age but persists into the ninth decade. Survival analysis

Fig. 3 The spectrum of obesity management. This diagram illustrates the broad range of overlapping activities which should be considered integral to obesity management.

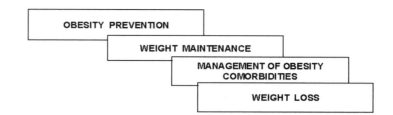

also reveals a highly elevated mortality risk in obese younger age groups linked to the duration of overweight[32]. This is clear evidence that concerted efforts should be made to prevent even modest weight gain in adults and in particular to control the weight of overweight children and young adults rather than allowing them to continue to increase their body weight with age[6,30].

The SIGN guidelines on the management of obesity in Scotland has highlighted the inappropriateness of separating prevention of obesity from other management strategies[13]. Indeed their definition of weight management includes the primary prevention of weight gain in children and adults, together with weight loss, weight maintenance and the management of weight-related risk factors (see Fig. 3). It has been estimated that without attention to preventive efforts, a general practice in the UK containing 10,000 patients would see an extra 80 patients becoming obese each year. Therefore, rather than avoiding the demand of time in prevention, failure to integrate obesity prevention in weight management strategies results in extra workload for all professionals within the health care system.

Areas of priority for preventive action

Deciding where to invest limited time and resources in effective obesity prevention is a difficult task but the prevention and effective management of overweight and obesity in children should be identified as a priority for action. Overweight and obesity during childhood is one of the major risk factors for the development of severe obesity in adulthood[10]; around 30% of obese children become obese adults. Furthermore, studies have shown that childhood obesity persisting into adulthood results in more severe obesity, with a higher morbidity and mortality rate, than adults whose obesity began in adulthood[23,33]. Childhood obesity also has immediate effects on health, including lowered fitness, orthopaedic problems, increased blood pressure and adverse blood lipid levels. Problems relating to psychosocial functioning are more common in obese children in Western societies, particularly during adolescence where self-awareness of body shape and appearance become more important[34].

A second area of priority for preventive action is undoubtedly that relating to public health or community-wide interventions. Although obesity prevention has not yet been explored in any depth amongst adults, attempts at long term weight loss or management have not proved encouraging. As a result the rates of overweight and obesity have risen dramatically in the UK over the last decade to the point where 57% of men and 48% of women[35] now have a BMI greater than 25 kg/m². Similar trends have been found in most developed and even in many developing countries[36]. Thus, obesity has clearly become one of the most important public health problems of the late 20th century and, as a result, preventive efforts must focus on the population as a whole. Adopting a public health approach to the prevention of obesity provides the best opportunity to tackle the problem of obesity in a coherent, logical fashion. Given the limited resources now available within health care systems, it is likely to be the most cost-effective approach. However, the effective implementation of public health approaches to the management of obesity will require a shift away from the traditional focus on clinical management and individual behaviour change towards strategies which deal with the environment in which such behaviours occur.

The remainder of this chapter will examine issues implicated in preventive approaches targeted at the two priority areas identified above: firstly the prevention of obesity during childhood; and secondly, a public health approach to obesity prevention.

Prevention of obesity during childhood

Special issues in the prevention of childhood obesity

There have so far been few controlled trials aimed at the prevention of obesity in children, and so most of our understanding in this area comes indirectly from analysis of treatment programmes for pre-existing childhood overweight and obesity.

The place of childhood obesity treatment in preventive efforts as outlined previously, the treatment of existing overweight and obesity during childhood can be regarded as a form of indicated prevention (Fig. 1) because childhood obesity increases the risk of adulthood obesity. Therefore, the treatment of childhood obesity should be considered along with selective prevention strategies aimed at high-risk groups of children and with universal approaches to the community-wide prevention of childhood obesity.

The objectives of weight management strategies for children differ from that for adults because consideration needs to be given to the physical and intellectual development of the child. Physical maturation places considerable nutritional demands on a child at a stage in life when they have limited capabilities to act independently. Therefore, whereas adult treatment may focus on weight loss, childhood treatment targets the prevention of weight gain. Children experience increases in lean body mass as they age, and so reducing or keeping fat mass constant can result in a normalisation of body weight.

Evidence to support the concept that treatment of childhood obesity prevents later adulthood obesity   the work of Epstein and colleagues[37] provides the most compelling evidence that the treatment of obesity in children can be successful over extended periods from childhood through adolescence to adulthood. In a series of four studies, 158 children were followed up, 10 years after their initial treatment. At the time of the initial treatment, the children had all been at high risk for significant adulthood obesity; they were 6–12 years of age, averaged 40–50% overweight, and had at least one obese parent. The studies investigated different treatment conditions, but all involved a diet plan together with group behaviour modification presented intensively over an 8–12 week period, followed by monthly maintenance sessions for 6–12 months.

Long-term results were encouraging; six out of nine actively treated groups showed a net reduction in percent overweight between 10–20%. The three remaining groups did not succeed long-term, but this was thought to be due to a lack of focus in the interventions offered to these groups.

Although it may be premature to make broad generalisations about the efficacy of obesity treatment in children, these studies give reason for optimism about the potential for comprehensive behavioural treatments to offer enduring benefits to obese children. A much needed research step is to conduct a longitudinal trial that evaluates whether results like those achieved by Epstein and colleagues can be replicated at other sites and in other populations, and whether tangible health benefits, both in health and social domains, can be demonstrated.

Objectives for preventive efforts

The analysis of childhood obesity management programmes has helped identify three factors which appear to be important intermediary behaviours in the development of obesity in children and, therefore, provide important foci for prevention efforts: a diet high in energy-dense foods and drinks and an absence of formal meals; lack of regular physical activity; and an inclination to pursue sedentary leisure pastimes.

Reducing energy intake in children an adequate intake of both energy and nutrients are required by a child for growth and development, and so excessive energy restriction in obese children is unwise and potentially unsafe. Thus, only a small reduction in energy intake is recommended and the overall diet must be varied and healthy.

One method of reducing energy intake in children is to limit portion sizes of energy-dense foods. Parents and other food providers can achieve this by preparing and serving smaller quantities of such foods, or by encouraging *ad libitum* consumption of fruits and vegetables so that energy-density is reduced without imposing dietary restriction. However, only limited data support the suggestion that an increased variety of food intake results in a decreased intake of energy dense foods[38].

Another way of restricting energy intake in children is to specifically limit foods that are high in dietary fat. Take-away and ready-prepared foods, which tend to be particularly high in fat and energy, are making increasingly larger contributions to the energy intake of children and adolescents in developed countries[39] and are an obvious target. Children should also be encouraged to eat fewer high-fat snacks such as crisps and biscuits, and to chose unsweetened drinks or water. However, one study on prepubertal children which attempted to reduce fat intake over 12 months did not achieve weight loss or reductions in weight gain within the target group despite achieving some dietary change[40].

Increasing regular physical activity in children children should be encouraged to be as active as possible. However, it appears that the primary goal should be to increase daily energy expenditure through general activity and play rather than through competitive sport and structured exercise[41]. Obese children have similar problems associated with adhering to long-term exercise programs as adults, and they are particularly sensitive to peer attitudes towards body shape and exercise performance. This tends to limit their willingness to be involved in team sports[42]. Increased energy expenditure is only one benefit of increased physical activity in children[43]. Therefore, the improvement of aerobic fitness should not be an overriding concern although this is likely to be another positive consequence. It is, therefore, unfortunate that attempts to improve the poor levels of physical activity in British schoolchildren have focused on the re-introduction of competitive sports.

Reducing inactivity in children the role of inactivity, or sedentary behaviour as it is more correctly described, in the genesis of children's weight problems has recently begun to attract more attention; particularly with the explosion of non-active leisure pursuits for children such as computers and video games. Television represents the principal source of inactivity for most children and adolescents in developed countries and long periods of viewing have been linked to the prevalence of obesity[44,45]. Television viewing is also associated with increased consumption of high energy snacks[31,45]. Of particular interest, a recent study by Epstein and others[106] clearly showed that short-term weight losses were greater in children who were instructed to reduce sedentary behaviour than in children who were encouraged to increase exercise. Reducing physical inactivity also resulted in improved maintenance of weight loss and a more positive attitude towards vigorous activity.

Obesity prevention strategies during childhood

Three key areas for action in the prevention and treatment of obesity during childhood have been shown to be of value in past interventions; initiating prevention through primary care, family-based support, and schools-based programmes. These are considered below.

Initiating prevention through primary care There has been little formal assessment of obesity prevention efforts through primary care, but its potential role appears to be under-valued and under-utilised[13]. As demonstrated by one general practitioner, the provision of healthy eating advice to pregnant women and their children restricted the rate of obesity within his patient sample to only 2% compared with levels closer to 8% in those patients who did not receive advice[46].

Health visitors and child health nurses play a crucial role in monitoring the development of infants and young children. Regular assessment and contact through home visits can provide valuable information concerning potential lifestyle risk factors for obesity as well as advice and support to help parents adopt healthy eating and exercise patterns at an early stage in life — before obesity develops. Davis and Christofel[11] found that early and frequent contact with health professionals was the most effective approach to the management of childhood obesity and thus similar strategies may be equally effective in prevention. It has been suggested that obesity prevention should start with appropriate advice about breastfeeding, weaning, and diet for toddlers[47].

Measuring fatness (or relative weight) in children is more complicated than equivalent assessments in adults because of the natural variations in adiposity with age throughout childhood. However, the recent development of BMI-for-age charts for UK children (birth to 23 years)[48] should make the monitoring of relative weight much simpler.

Family-based programmes The family environment can strongly influence a child's risk of obesity; parental attitudes, purchase and presentation of food, parental modelling of eating and exercise habits, and support for active leisure pursuits can all effect a child's eating and exercise pattern. Providing appropriate eating and lifestyle behaviour education to parents has been shown to reduce the prevalence of obesity in children of participating families for periods of 3 months to 3 years when compared to families not receiving advice and support[49]. By directing obesity preventive efforts at the family of susceptible children there is the added bonus that all members of the family are likely to benefit.

A number of successful childhood obesity and weight management programmes have provided strong evidence for the important role of family support in such interventions. Epstein and colleagues[50] suggested that weight regulation effects are improved if at least one parent is included with the child in treatment. When they compared the effect of targeting an overweight child alone with that of targeting a child and a parent together, the latter group showed significantly less weight gain at 5 years follow-up and were still below the relative weight at which they started the study at 10 years follow-up (Fig. 4A). This finding is even more significant as maintenance of relative weight occurred throughout adolescence when weight gain can be a problem. These trials also suggested that children of non-obese parents were better able to obtain and maintain reductions in relative weight (Fig. 4B). Other investigators have also found improved effectiveness of family based programmes in preventing the progression of childhood obesity. Flodmark *et al.*[9] found improved weight loss or maintenance in children (aged 10–11 years) treated with family therapy when compared to those treated alone. Similar findings were made by Wadden and others[51] in black American teenage girls.

The success of involving at least one parent in the management of childhood weight problems has been associated with the increased social support and reduction in the feeling of isolation that may occur when one child is treated separately from the rest of the family. Parents are also able to exert a higher degree of external control over the child's eating and activity patterns under these circumstances[52].

School based programmes The school is an extremely important and useful site for instituting obesity prevention programmes since a large proportion of all children attend school and a great deal of a child's

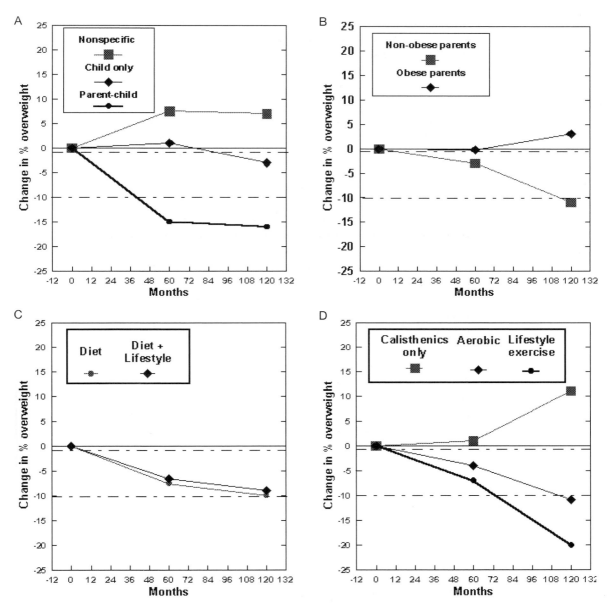

Fig. 4 Changes in percentage overweight after 5 and 10 years follow-up for obese children randomly assigned to ten interventions across four studies. The results of four separate studies in which Epstein et al.[50] examined the impact of different interventions for obesity management in overweight children. All studies had the same basic diet and behaviour change intervention over 8–12 weeks with monthly review for 6–12 months together with the additional element under investigation. Study A compared involving children alone, children and a parent or no specific directions. Study B compared relative weight changes in children of obese and non-obese parents. Study C examined the benefit of adding lifestyle exercise to a diet programme and study D compared the effectiveness of different forms of exercise in aiding weight control. The children and parents were followed up 5 years and 10 years after the initial programme. The results show excellent long term benefits and demonstrate the value of family support and the value of a positive family environment and the value of unstructured (lifestyle) exercise in weight control for children. The 95% confidence interval for the total sample of children is represented by dotted lines. [Source: Epstein et al. (1994) ©American Psychological Association. Reprinted with permission.]

eating and exercise is carried out in this setting. Furthermore, starting school coincides with a period of increased risk for excessive weight gain as children begin to exert independence and vary their diet and activity patterns in line with their new circumstance. The downgrading of the school medical service within the UK and a number of other countries is unfortunate as regular assessments at key developmental stages by a school doctor or nurse can help identify children who may be at risk of obesity. These health professionals can also establish or contribute to school-based educational or support programmes for overweight children.

Results from various school-based obesity intervention programmes which have targeted high-risk children and adolescents suggest that these can be successfully implemented and can reach substantial numbers of children in need of obesity prevention[53–55]. Obese children in treatment groups have consistently shown greater reductions in percent overweight than untreated obese controls. Results over periods of 3–6 months are modestly encouraging and justify additional research in this area.

Increasing physical activity through integrating regular exercise programmes into school curricula is a strategy that has often been proposed as an effective means of improving weight and health status of children[16,56]. The evaluation of a 2 year project in South Australia, where 50 min of daily physical activity was introduced into a number of primary schools demonstrated that children who took part in the programme were fitter, slimmer, had lower diastolic blood pressure (boys only), than their non participating counterparts[57]. A subsequent study which built on this project by including classroom lessons on nutrition and physical health was also able to demonstrate improvements in indices of fitness and body fat levels[58]. Similar programmes have also been run in US[43] and Singapore schools[59] where short term results are promising. Despite demonstrating positive benefits, the maintenance of these programmes within the school curricula in the long term has proved more difficult due to competition for school time, the need for teacher/adult supervision and financial limitations.

Points of caution

The value of prudent attempts to prevent excessive weight gain in normal weight children or to reduce weight gain in children who are already obese is apparent. However, it should be emphasised that care must be taken in developing interventions aimed at preventing or treating obesity in young children. Firstly, as adequate nutrition is essential for promoting healthy growth, only small reductions in overall energy intake are recommended where such an approach is advised. Secondly, it is important that interventions do not encourage the type of dietary restraint that has been linked to the development of eating disorders and other forms of psychological distress[52]. Finally, it is also very important that overweight children are not ostracised and made to feel any more different than is necessary either at home or at school[33]. The message that everyone is potentially at risk of obesity may help but there is also a need to generate family awareness of the need for healthier lifestyles without suggesting that the goal is to lose weight.

A public health approach to obesity prevention

The principles

Public health deals with health problems from a population or community perspective and is sometimes viewed as confused and unfocussed by health professionals who are more used to the idea of caring for, and improving the health of, individuals. However, health problems which impact upon the well-being of a major proportion of the population are unlikely to be effectively controlled by strategies that focus on disparate individuals. Public health action is based on the principle that promoting and protecting the health of the population requires an integrated approach encompassing environmental, educational, economic, technical and legislative measures together with a health care system oriented to the early detection and management of disease[60].

A public health approach to obesity attempts to shift the focus of action away from strategies which deal exclusively with those factors influencing body fatness of individuals and towards strategies dealing with the weight status of the population as a whole.

Why intervene at the population level?

Whilst there is widespread acknowledgement of the important role of public health action in the control of infectious disease, there is still some scepticism concerning the applicability of this approach to the management of non-infectious diseases such as CHD and obesity. Some observers have questioned the merit of population level interventions because all members of the community may be required to make changes (or have them imposed upon them) to deal with a problem that currently affects only a proportion of those individuals[14,61,62]. However, if the link

A

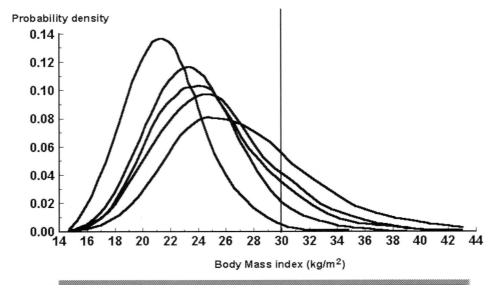

The shifting distributions of BMI of five population groups of men and women aged 20-59 years derived from 52 surveys in 32 countries.

B

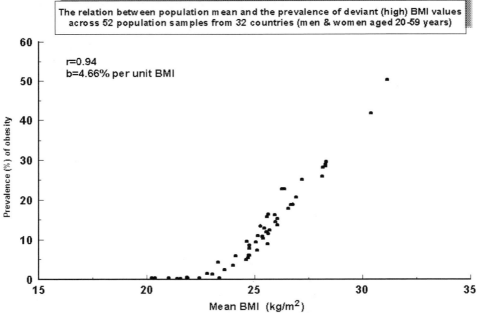

The relation between population mean and the prevalence of deviant (high) BMI values across 52 population samples from 32 countries (men & women aged 20-59 years)

Fig. 5 The relationship between population mean BMI and the level of obesity. These two analyses of body weight data from 52 communities in the INTERSALT study by Rose[63] show the clear relationship between population mean BMI and the level of obesity in population. As the mean population BMI increases the level of obesity increases at an even faster rate because of the skewing of the distribution to higher BMIs. Public health interventions aim to prevent this upward shift in mean population BMI. [Source: Rose (1991) ©Springer–Verlag. Reproduced with permission.]

between the average and extreme levels of body fatness within a population (Fig. 5A,B) is understood, then the importance of population level interventions in obesity can be appreciated.

The relationship between average population BMI and the level of obesity obesity in adults is usually classified as a BMI > 30 kg/m². However, this is a purely arbitrary figure indicating greatly increased health risks at this level of body fatness and does not imply that BMIs below this level are free from associated risks. It is, therefore, not appropriate to consider the population as two distinct groups, the 'obese' and the 'non-obese' when, in practice, the distribution of body fatness of individuals in a population is continuous ranging from underweight through normal to very obese and the risks of associated morbidity and mortality begin at relatively low levels of BMI.

An analysis of body weight data from 52 communities in the multi-country INTERSALT study by Rose[63] was able to demonstrate variations in the distribution of BMI in different populations that could be predicted from the population mean BMI. When the average BMI of a population is in the range 20–22 kg/m² there are few, if any, individuals with a BMI > 30 kg/m². But, as the BMI distribution of the community shifts to the right (i.e. mean BMI increases), there is an increased skew and a flattening of the curve (Fig. 4A); which results in a greater number of individuals in the population whose BMI exceeds 30 kg/m². But, more importantly, the proportion of adults classified as obese increases at an even faster rate than the average BMI. Rose found that there is a 4.66% increase in the prevalence of obesity for every single unit increase in the population's average BMI above 23 kg/m². This results in a strong correlation between the average adult BMI of a population and the proportion of adults with obesity (Fig. 4B). In the UK the mean BMI has increased from 24.3 kg/m² and 23.9 kg/m² for men and women, respectively, in 1980 to 29.9 kg/m² and 25.7 kg/m², in 1993. Yet, over this same period, the rate of overweight has increased by a third whilst obesity rates have doubled in both men and women. This implies that further increases in mean BMI are likely to result in even more dramatic rises in the rates of obesity.

From the above, it can be seen that effective prevention of obesity should focus on preventing the rise in the mean BMI of the community. Focusing obesity prevention and management efforts on people with existing weight problems (individuals in the right hand tail of the distribution in Fig. 4A) will do little to reduce the increasingly larger proportions of the population who enter the high risk categories for weight if the mean population BMI continues to increase.

Public health interventions

There are generally two types of public health intervention strategy that can be used to tackle obesity: (i) those which aim to improve the knowledge and skills of individuals in a community; and (ii) those which aim to reduce exposure of populations to the underlying environmental causes of obesity.

Improving the knowledge and skills of the community To date, virtually all public health interventions aimed at the population control of obesity have been from an individual perspective. They have generally relied on education and behaviour-change strategies that can be disseminated to a wide audience; through mass-media education, worksite interventions, school-based programs and education curricula, skills training delivered within a network of clubs and community centres, and multi-strategy community projects.

In contrast to many other public health problems, however, strategies aimed at improving the knowledge and skills of the community have not produced impressive results in dealing with obesity. This may be because communities are already generally well aware of the problems associated with obesity and many individuals are already actively attempting to control their weight. Participation rates are usually high and many succeed in reducing their weight, at least in the short-term. However, there is generally little impact on the average BMI of the community and only a negligible effect on obesity prevalence[64].

The apparent failure of public health interventions that have attempted to control population obesity from an individual perspective is not a reason for abandoning such approaches. Instead, it illustrates the need to review the effectiveness of these strategies when they are delivered in isolation, i.e. without attending to the other more powerful societal and environmental obesity-promoting influences.

Reducing population exposure to an obesity-promoting environment A more effective strategy for dealing with the public health problem of obesity would appear to be one that goes beyond the educational dimension, and deals with those environmental and societal factors that induce the obesity-promoting behaviour of individuals within a population in the first place. In this way, we may reduce the exposure of the whole population to obesity-promoting forces such as the persistent temptation of high-fat foods, and the convenience of a sedentary lifestyle. Unfortunately, however, strategies such as these remain relatively unexplored.

Past public health interventions in controlling obesity

There have not, to date, been any well-evaluated and truly concerted public health programmes aimed at the population-level management or prevention of obesity. A number of countries have recently developed a lifestyle strategy with a focus on weight control but these have not been set up as controlled trials and so are unlikely to provide any definitive evidence of their impact.

The nearest examples that we have are community-wide coronary heart disease prevention programmes that have included a reduction in BMI as one of the measurable outcomes. The Stanford Three Community Project[65], the Stanford Five City Study[66] and the Minnesota Heart Health Program[67] all utilised mass media, interpersonal education, and community organisation to increase awareness and knowledge about CHD and to teach skills required for appropriate behaviour change to reduce CHD risk. In depth evaluation of these programmes and their results revealed that, although significant reductions were achieved in many CHD risk factors, only very small improvements were seen in body weight. The North Karelia Project[68] and the Mauritius Non-communicable Diseases Intervention Project[69] both involved wide-spread community participation but also found obesity harder to control than any other risk factor.

Other controlled trials have investigated the potential to positively influence factors identified as important in the development of obesity, such as physical activity and the quality of the food supply. Evaluation of these programmes suggests that intensive community-wide intervention can improve physical activity participation rates, at least in the short term, but the long term maintenance of increased physical activity and its potential benefits on obesity prevention remain unproved[70,71]. Reductions in dietary fat intake of the population have been more difficult to achieve within the short time frames associated with most studies. However, Norway and Finland have instituted broad reaching national nutrition programmes and have been able to reduce national fat intake from 42% to 34% of total dietary energy over the last 20 years. It is, therefore, encouraging to see that the increase in obesity prevalence is slowing in Finland and the mean BMI is stabilising despite concomitant decreases in physical activity levels[72]. A recent study which analysed data from all 40–42 year old men and women recruited to a country-wide CHD prevention programme throughout Norway (except Oslo) indicated that obesity rates have decreased slightly in females since the 1960s[73]. However, they have increased substantially in men over the same period but still remain lower than other European countries.

Possible explanations as to why most of these community-wide intervention programmes have been disappointing in terms of obesity and weight control have been suggested by Jeffery[74]. He points out that these programmes were based on personal education and behaviour change in older age groups without attempting to influence the environmental factors — such as transportation, urban design, advertising, food pricing, etc. — which impact upon our food choices and daily activity patterns. Exalting people to change their behaviours to improve the quality of their diet and their physical activity level is unlikely to succeed in an environment in which there are plentiful inducements to engage in opposing behaviours that lead to a chronic positive energy imbalance.

Country-wide public health obesity programmes At present there are very few countries that have a comprehensive population-wide national policy or strategy to deal specifically with the problem of overweight and obesity. This is despite reports being produced within a number a countries such as Australia[75], Canada[76], and the UK[77] which have all indicated that this is precisely what is required to tackle obesity effectively.

Singapore is one country that has been able to achieve a degree of success in tackling obesity through a system of co-ordinated healthy lifestyle programmes aimed at specific target groups across the population. The Government of Singapore has an overall strategy which is translated into programmes directed at all stages of life including pre-school, school years, national service and broader community projects for adults. Such programmes rely heavily on input from the community in their establishment and ongoing management[59]. The *Trim and Fit* programme which was launched in 1992 is aimed at all schoolchildren in Singapore and combines progressive nutrition changes in school catering and nutrition education with regular physical activity within schools. This is supported by specialised training for school principals, teachers and tuckshop workers, as well as the provision of equipment for improved catering and physical activity. A national monitoring programme to assess fitness and weight status also runs in conjunction with this initiative[78]. Recent results indicate that the number of children successfully completing the fitness tests is improving annually and that the rates of obesity have dropped from 14.3% in 1992 to 10.9% in 1996 for primary students, 14.1% to 10.9% for secondary students and 10.8% to 6.1% for junior college students[79].

Lessons to be learned form other successful public health campaigns

Public health programmes to manage obesity are unlikely to achieve the same spectacular rates of success as those in the past associated with the control of infectious disease. Unlike the case of pathogens, it is not feasible to remove totally the cause of obesity. Nor is it a simple process to isolate and manage exposure to a single major obesity-promoting contributory factor as has been the case with certain other non-communicable diseases. Control of smoking and hypertension, for instance, have contributed greatly to the successful reduction in rates of CHD. However, analysis of the features of other relatively successful public health campaigns such as those to address smoking, seat belt wearing, drink driving and immunisation has helped identify character-istics of these campaigns that may provide important leads for public health interventions to control obesity.

- A consistent and important feature of all successful public health campaigns aimed at behaviour change is the time required to see the impact of any intervention and the need for persistency is continuing campaigns. Changes in CHD risk factors were unspectacular in the first 10 years of the campaign in Finland, but improvements have accelerated in recent years[80].
- A change in behaviour is not a unitary event but a process with a number of stages. It is unrealistic to expect rapid change in complex behaviours, such as eating and exercise, when even changing a single behaviour, such as cigarette smoking, has been shown to require a series of strategies over time which support the transition from awareness, through motivation, to change, experimenting and adopting a change to maintenance of that behaviour change[81].
- Gains in seat-belt wearing and drink driving have only been achieved with legislative support. Attitudinal and behaviour shifts occurred after legisla-tive change rather than preceding or directing changes in regulations[82].
- The need for systematic co-ordinated approach which includes education as well as regulation is highlighted in improvements in immunisation rates for many childhood diseases. Education can encourage and support a change in behaviour and avoid the feeling that change is being imposed without reason[83].
- The need for strong advocacy from respected elements within all sections of society has been a key feature of the improvement in smoking rates and exposure to passive cigarette smoke. Although healthcare workers are highly regarded within most communities, opinion leaders and role models tend to come from other sectors of society[68].

Potential public health strategies to improve the prevention and management of obesity

Obesity is a complex and poorly understood disease. Its aetiology is the product of an interaction of genetic, biological and environmental factors. However, the fact that recent dramatic rises in the rates of obesity have occurred in such a short time frame and within the same genetic pool suggest that biological factors are not the basis for the escalating problem of obesity today. Nor does it seem feasible that a sudden breakdown in personal control is responsible for a doubling of obesity rates in the UK in the last 15 years. Yet many people persist in believing that the problem of obesity is a consequence of poor personal behaviours; the product of gluttony and sloth. This bias against obese people and an over-emphasis of personal responsibility has resulted in the key role of the environment in the development of obesity being largely ignored.

Most developed countries have created an environment that is highly conducive to a positive energy balance. High fat, energy dense, appealing food is more readily available than ever before. It is packaged attractively, requires little or no preparation, is advertised heavily using questionable tactics and is relatively cheap. A recent survey of advertising on television in the UK[84] revealed that 70% of advertisements during peak children's viewing time were for food products and that between 90–100% of these food items could be classed as either high in fat, sugar and/or salt using the classification system of the Coronary Prevention Group. In addition, there is an imbalance in promotional messages children receive; in the UK, for example, £80 million was spent on promoting the consumption of chocolate in 1992, whilst only £3 million was spent on promoting the consumption of vegetables and fruit[85]. The number of fast food outlets in the UK more than doubled in the ten years between 1984–93, whilst the number of traditional eating places fell[85]. It is not surprising that purchasing a low energy meal or snack from some catering outlets or canteens is often a frustrating and difficult task.

Television viewing has become the major leisure pursuit of children and adults. Research from the US and Canada reveals that children aged 10–15 years watch, on average, 34 h of television per week and younger children watch even more[86]. Recent surveys indicate that involvement in leisure time activity may be increasing but the intensity of that activity is decreasing[87] and participation is often limited by the availability and cost of using facilities. The level of occupational activity has also been declining, with a shift in composition of the labour force to more sedentary professions. Between 1985–92, the average distance walked by English children (14 years and younger) decreased by 20%, the average distance cycled decreased by 25%, while distance travelled by car increased by 40%[107]. Furthermore, whilst road networks expand there has been little investment in cycle paths. Buildings are designed on the assumption that lifts are preferable to the use of stairs and there is a common perception that it is unsafe to walk or play in the streets due to the risk posed by traffic or crime.

Table 3 Potential environmental strategies to control obesity

Area for action	Example of potential strategies
Urban design and transportation policies	● Construction of safe walkways and cycle paths ● Improved lighting for safe walking ● Traffic calming to improve safety for children walking and playing ● Community recreation centres ● Improved building design to encourage use of stairs
Regulation and legislation	● Improved labelling of food products ● Limits on advertising to children ● Regulation to ensure that vegetables or salad are served at no extra cost with every meal sold from certain food outlets
Economic incentives	● Subsidies for producers of low energy dense foods (especially fruit and vegetables) ● Reduced car tax on those who take public transport to work during the week ● Tax breaks for companies that provide exercise and change facilities for employers
Improved catering standards and food preparation skills	● Nutrition standards for school meals and worksite catering ● Improved training in practical food skills for all school children
Education and promotion	● Improved education of the community on the development of obesity to reduce victimisation of the obese ● Education on appropriate behaviour change to reduce risk of weight gain, especially in areas where food is purchased ● Education on the need for collective action to improve our environment so that it promotes rather than inhibits improved exercise and diet habits

In the face of this environment, it is not surprising that interventions that have focused on education for behaviour change have had limited success in controlling obesity. There is a desperate need to refocus obesity prevention efforts to ensure greater attention to producing an environment which supports improved eating and physical activity habits throughout the entire community. This will require a comprehensive and integrated range of strategies in line with the examples set out in Table 3. The implementation of such an approach will require the acceptance that the management of obesity is not just the responsibility of individuals, their families or health professionals but requires a commitment from all sectors of society. Until this is achieved, the effective prevention and management of obesity will remain problematic.

Key points for clinical practice

Obesity is a serious medical condition associated with a wide range of chronic and debilitating conditions. Obesity develops over time and once developed is difficult to treat. Therefore, prevention of weight gain offers the only truly effective means of controlling obesity.

Although obese patients will have a markedly higher risk of certain illnesses and death, the association between weight and ill health begins to increase steadily from a body mass index of less than 20 kg/m² and the extent of ill health is directly related to the duration of overweight. Therefore, regular monitoring of BMI should be undertaken with every patient and concerted efforts should be made to control even modest weight gains in adults. Prevention of weight gain should be considered an integral component of all obesity management protocols together with weight maintenance, management of obesity comorbidities and weight loss where appropriate.

Particular attention should be paid to weight management at certain vulnerable ages and life-stages and in certain groups of patients who are at increased risk of developing obesity due to genetic, social, or behavioural factors.

The prevention and management of overweight and obesity in children is particularly important as one-third of obese children become obese adults. However, caution must be exercised as childhood is a stage of rapid physical, psychological and social development that can be compromised by vigorous intervention. Involvement of the whole family in any weight management efforts improves success rates and prevents individual children being ostracised. Health professionals have an important role in monitoring children's weight and advising and supporting diet and lifestyle change to prevent the development of weight problems. BMI for age charts have recently been published for use with British children.

Obesity is a population problem and needs to be tackled at a population level with input from all sectors of society. Effective prevention of obesity will require public health programmes that deal with the societal and environmental factors that are conducive to reduced physical activity or increased energy intake. The establishment of such programmes will require the advocacy and support of the medical profession.

Acknowledgements

I would like to thank Philip James for his advice and the staff of the Post Graduate Nutrition and Dietetic Centre at the Rowett Research Institute for their assistance in the development and production of this article.

References

1 Garner DM, Wooley SC. Confronting the failure of behavioural and dietary treatments for obesity. *Clin Psychol Rev* 1991; 11: 573–8
2 Weintraub M, Sundaresan PR, Schuster B. Long term weight control: the National Heart, Lung and Blood Institute-funded multimodal intervention study. I–VII. *Clin Pharmacol Ther* 1992; 51: 581–646

3 Kayman S, Bruvold W, Stern JS. Maintenance and relapse after weight loss in women: behavioural aspects. *Am J Clin Nutr* 1990; **52**: 800–7

4 Pi-Sunyer FX. Medical aspects of obesity. *Ann Intern Med* 1993; **119**: 655–60

5 Higgins M, D'Agostino R, Kannel W, Cobb J. Benefits and adverse effects of weight loss: observations from the Framingham Study. *Ann Intern Med* 1993; **119**: 758–63

6 James WPT. The epidemiology of obesity. In: *The origins and consequences of obesity*. Ciba Foundation Symposium 201. Chichester: Wiley, 1996; 1–16

7 Forster JL, Jeffery RW, Schmidt TL, Kramer M. Preventing weight gain in adults. A pound of prevention. *Health Psychol* 1988; **7**: 515–25

8 Epstein LH, Valoski A, Wing RR, McCurley J. Ten-year outcomes of behavioural family-based treatment for childhood obesity. *Health Psychol* 1994; **13**: 373–83

9 Flodmark C-E, Ohlsson T, Ryden O, Sveger T. Prevention of progression to severe obesity in a groups of obese schoolchildren treated with family therapy. *Pediatrics* 1993; **91**: 880–4

10 Dietz HW. Therapeutic strategies in childhood obesity. *Hormone Res* 1993; **39** (**Suppl 3**): 86–90

11 Davis K, Christoffel KK. Obesity in preschool and school-age children: treatment early and often is best. *Arch Pediatr Adolesc Med* 1994; **148**: 1257–61

12 US Institute of Medicine. *Reducing risks for mental disorders: frontiers for preventative intervention research*. Report of the Committee on Prevention of Medical Disorders. Division of Biobehavioural Sciences and Mental Disorders. Washington: National Academy Press, 1994

13 SIGN (Scottish Intercollegiate Guidelines Network). *Obesity in Scotland. Integrating prevention with weight management*. Edinburgh: HMSO, 1996

14 Oliver MF. Should we not forget about mass control of coronary risk factors? *Lancet* 1983; **2**: 37–8

15 Stunkard AJ. Prevention of obesity. In: Brownell KD, Fairburn CG (eds) *Eating Disorders and Obesity. A Comprehensive Handbook*. London: Guilford Press, 1995; 572–6

16 James WPT. A public health approach to the problem of obesity. *Int J Obes* 1995: **19** (**Suppl 3**): 37S–45S

17 Bray GA. To treat or not to treat. In: Bray GA (ed) *Recent Advances in Obesity Research* vol 11. London: Newman Publishing, 1978

18 Waaler HT. Height, weight and mortality: the Norwegian experience. *Acta Med Scand* 1984; **679**: 1–56

19 Simopoulis AP, van Itallie TB. Body weight, health and longevity. *Ann Intern Med* 1984; **100**: 285–90

20 Hall A, Franz CP. Obesity: time for sanity and humanity. *N Z Med J* 1989; **102**: 134

21 Wooley SC, Garner DM. Obesity treatment: the high cost of false hope. *J Am Diet Assoc* 1991; **91**: 1248–51

22 Manson JE, Stampfer MJ, Hennekens CH, Willett WC. Body weight and longevity: a reassessment. *JAMA* 1987; **257**: 353–8

23 Seidell JC, Verschuren M, van Leer EM *et al*. Overweight, underweight and mortality: a prospective study of 48,287 men and women. *Arch Intern Med* 1996; **156**: 958–63

24 Manson JE, Willey WC, Stampfer MJ *et al*. Body weight and mortality among women. *N Engl J Med* 1995; **333**: 677–85

25 Linsted K, Tonstad S, Kusma JW. Body mass index and patterns of mortality among Seventh-day Adventist men. *Int J Obes* 1991; **15**: 397–406

26 Chan JM, Rimm EB, Colditz GA, Stampfer MJ, Willet WC. Obesity, fat distribution and weight gain as risk factors for clinical diabetes in men. *Diabetes Care* 1994; **17**: 961–9

27 Rissanen A, Heliövaara M, Knekt P, Reunanen A, Maatela J. Risk of disability and mortality in a Finnish population. *BMJ* 1990; **30**: 835–7

28 Shaper AG. Obesity and cardiovascular disease. In: *The Origins and Consequences of Obesity*. Ciba Foundation Symposium 201. Chichester: Wiley, 1996; 90–107

29 Blackburn GL, Dwyer J, Flanders WD *et al*. Report of the American Institute of Nutrition (AIN) Steering Committee on Healthy Weight. *J Nutr* 1994; **124**: 2240–3

30 Garrow JS. *Treat Obesity Seriously: A Clinical Manual*. Edinburgh: Churchill Livingstone, 1982

31 Dietz HW. Prevention of childhood obesity. *Pediatr Clin North Am* 1986; **33**: 823–33

32 Must A, Jacques PF, Dallal GE, Bajema CJ, Dietz WH. Long term morbidity and mortality of overweight adolescents. *N Eng J Med* 1992; **327**; 1350–5

33 Dietz HW. Childhood obesity. In: Bjorntrop P, Brodoff BN (eds) *Obesity*. Philadelphia: Lippincott, 1992; 606–9

34 French SA, Story M, Perry CL. Self-esteem and obesity in children and adolescents: a literature review. *Obes Res* 1995; **3**: 479–90

35 Bennett N, Dodd T, Flatley J, Freeth S, Bolling K. *Health Survey for England 1993*. Series HS no 3. London: HMSO, 1995

36 Seidell JC. Obesity in Europe — scaling an epidemic. *Int J Obes* 1995; **19 (Suppl 3)**: S1–S4

37 Epstein LH, Valoski A, Wing RR, McCurley J. Ten-year follow-up of behavioural, family-based treatment for obese children. *JAMA* 1990; **264**: 2519–23

38 Kennedy E, Goldberg J. What are American children eating? Implications for public policy. *Nutr Rev* 1995; **53**: 111–26

39 McKenzie J. Social changes and the food industry. *Nutr Rev* 1982; **40 (Suppl)**: 13–7

40 DISC Collaborative Research Group. Efficacy and safety of lowering dietary intake of fat and cholesterol in children with elevated lipoprotein cholesterol: the Dietary Intervention Study in Children (DISC). *JAMA* 1995; **273**: 1429–35

41 Epstein LH, Wing RR, Koeske R, Valoski A. A comparison of lifestyle exercise, aerobic exercise and callisthenics on weight loss in obese children. *Behav Ther* 1985; **16**: 345–6

42 Court JM. Strategies for the management of obesity in children and adolescents. In: Hills AP, Wahlqvist ML, (eds) *Exercise and Obesity*. London: Smith Gordon, 1994; 181–95

43 Epstein LH. Exercise in the treatment of childhood obesity. *Int J Obes* 1995; **19**: 117S–121S

44 Dietz WH, Gortmaker SL. Do we fatten our children at the television set? Obesity and television viewing in children and adolescents. *Pediatrics* 1985; **75**: 807–12

45 Gortmaker SL, Dietz HW, Cheung LW. Inactivity, diet and the fattening of America. *J Am Diet Assoc* 1990; **90**: 1247–52

46 Craddock D. *Obesity and its Management* 3rd edn. Edinburgh: Churchill Livingstone, 1978; 160–73

47 Leung AK, Robson WL. Childhood obesity. *Postgrad Med* 1990; **87**: 123–30

48 Cole TJ, Freeman JV, Preece MA. Body mass index curves for the UK. *Arch Dis Child* 1995; **73**: 25–9

49 Pisacano JC, Lichter H, Ritter J, Siegal AP. An attempt at prevention of obesity in infancy. *Pediatrics* 1978; **61**: 360–4

50 Epstein LH, Valoski A, Wing RR, McCurley J. Ten-year outcomes of behavioural family-based treatment for childhood obesity. *Health Psychol* 1994; **13**: 373–83

51 Wadden TA, Stunkard AJ, Rich L *et al*. Obesity in black adolescent girls: a controlled clinical trial of treatment by diet, behaviour modification and parental support. *Pediatrics* 1990; **85**: 345–52

52 Wilson GT. Behavioural treatment of childhood obesity: theoretical and practical implications. *Health Psychol* 1994; **13**: 371–2

53 Seltzer CC, Mayer J. An effective weight control program in a public school system. *Am J Public Health* 1970; **60**: 679–89

54 Forster GD, Wadden TA, Brownell KD. Peer-led program for the treatment and prevention of children in schools. *J Consult Clin Psychol* 1985; **53**: 538–40

55 Resnicow K. School-based obesity prevention: population versus high risk interventions. *Ann NY Acad Sci* 1993; **699**: 154–66

56 Sleap N, Warburton P. *Physical Activity Patterns of Primary Schoolchildren: An Interim Report*. London: Health Education Authority, 1990

57 Dwyer T, Coonan WE, Leitch DR, Hetzel BS, Baghurst PA. An investigation of the effects of daily physical activity on health of primary school students in South Australia. *Int J Epidemiol* 1983; **12**: 308–13

58 Worsley A, Coonan W, Worsely A. The first body owner's programme: an integrated school-based physical and nutrition education programme. *Health Promotion* 1987; **2**: 39–49

59 Rajan U. Management of childhood obesity — Singapore perspective. *Proc MASSO* 1996; **1**: 131–7

60   Committee of enquiry into the future development of public health function. *Public Health in England*. London: HMSO, 1988

61   Atrens DM. The questionable wisdom of a low-fat diet and cholesterol reduction. *Soc Sci Med* 1994; **39**: 433–47

62   McCormick J, Srabanek P. Coronary heart disease is not preventable by population interventions. *Lancet* 1988; **2**: 839–41

63   Rose G. Population distributions of risk and disease. *Nutr Metab Cardiovasc Dis* 1991; **1**: 37–40

64   Jeffery RW. Public health approaches to the management of obesity. In: Brownell KD, Fairburn CG (eds) *Eating Disorders and Obesity. A Comprehensive Handbook*. London: Guilford Press, 1995; 558–63

65   Fortmann SP, Williams PT, Hulley SB *et al*. Effect of health education on dietary behaviors: the Stanford Three Community Study. *Am J Clin Nutr* 1981; **34**: 2030–8

66   Barr-Taylor C, Fortmann SP, Flora J *et al*. Effect of long-term community health education on body mass index. *Am J Epidemiol* 1991; **134**: 235–49

67   Jeffery RW, Gray CW, French SA *et al*. Evaluation of weight reduction in a community intervention for cardiovascular disease risk: changes in body mass index in the Minnesota Heart Health Program. *Int J Obes* 1995: **19**: 1173–8

68   Puska P, Nissinen A, Tuomilehto J *et al*. The community-based strategy to prevent coronary heart disease: conclusions from the ten years of the North Karelia Project. *Annu Rev Public Health* 1985; **6**: 147–93

69   Dowse GK, Gareeboo H, Alberti KGMM *et al*. Changes in population cholesterol concentrations and other cardiovascular risk factor levels after five years of the non-communicable disease intervention programme in Mauritius. *BMJ* 1995; **311**: 1255–9

70   King AC. Community intervention for promotion of physical activity and fitness. *Exerc Sport Sci Rev* 1991; **19**: 211–559

71   Owen N, Bauman A, Booth M, Oldenburg B, Magnus P. Serial mass-media campaigns to promote physical activity — reinforcing or redundant. *Am J Public Health* 1995; **85**: 244–8

72   Pietinen P, Vartiainen E, Männisto S. Trends in body mass index and obesity among adults in Finland from 1972 to 1992. *Int J Obes* 1996; **20**: 114–20

73   Tverdal A. Height, weight and body mass index for men and women aged 40–42 years. *Tidsskr Nor Loegeforen* 1996; **116**: 2152–6

74   Jeffery RW. Community programs for obesity prevention: the Minnesota Heart Health Program. *Obes Res* 1995; **3**: 283S–288S

75   ASSO (Australian Society for the Study of Obesity). *Healthy Weight Australia – A National Strategy*. Sydney: ASSO, 1995

76   Health and Welfare. Health Services and Promotion Branch, Health and Welfare Canada. *Promoting Healthy Weights: A Discussion Paper*. Ottawa: Minister of Supply and Services, Canada, 1988

77   HON. Nutrition and Physical Activity Task Force, The Health of the Nation. *Obesity; Reversing the Increasing Problem of Obesity in England*. London: Department of Health, 1995

78   Ministry of Education, Singapore. *The National Healthy Lifestyle Programme, Singapore* 1994

79   Ministry of Education, Singapore. *Update on Trim and Fit Programme*. 1996

80   Vartiaitnen E, Puska P, Jousilahti P *et al*. Twenty-year trends in coronary heart risk factors in North Karelia and in other areas of Finland. *Int J Epidemiol* 1994; **23**: 495–504

81   Borland R, Owen N, Hill DJ, Chapman S. Regulatory innovations, behaviour and health: implications of research on workplace smoking bans. *Int Rev Health Psychol* 1994; **3**: 167–85

82   Reynolds C. Legislation and the new public health. *Community Health Studies* 1989; **XIII**: 397–402

83   LeFebvre CR, Flora JA. Social marketing and public health intervention. *Health Educ Q* 1988; **15**: 219–315

84   Dibb S, Castwell A. *Easy to Swallow, Hard to Stomach: the Results of a Survey of Food Advertising on Television*. London: The National Food Alliance, 1995

85   Keynote Publications. *Keynote Market Research: Industry Trends and Forecasts UK Food Market* 4th edn. London: Keynote Publications, 1992

86 Pate RP, Long BJ, Heath G. Descriptive epidemiology of physical activity in adolescents. *Paediatr Exerc Sci* 1994; **6**: 434–7

87 *Allied Dunbar National Fitness Survey*. London: The Health Education Authority and Sports Council, 1992

88 Jackson AA, Langley-Evans SC, McCarthy HD. Nutritional influences in early life upon obesity and body proportions. In: *The Origins and Consequences of Obesity*. Ciba Foundation Symposium 201. Chichester: Wiley, 1996; 118–29

89 Rolland-Cachera MF, Deheeger M, Bellisle F *et al.* Adiposity rebound in children: a simple indicator for predicting obesity in children. *Am J Clin Nutr* 1984; **39**: 129–35

90 Dietz W. Critical periods in childhood for the development of obesity. *Am J Clin Nutr* 1994; **59**: 955–9

91 Wing R. Changing diet and exercise behaviours in individuals at risk of weight gain. *Obes Res* 1995; **3** (**Suppl 2**): 277S–282S

92 Ohlin A, Rossner S. Maternal body weight development after pregnancy. *Int J Obes* 1990; **14**: 159–73

93 The writing group for the PEPI trial. Effects of estrogen or estrogen/progestin regimens on heart disease risk factors in post menopausal women. The Postmenopausal Estrogen/Progestin Interventions (PEPI) trial. *JAMA* 1995; **273**: 199–208

94 Bouchard C. (ed) *The Genetics of Obesity*. Boca Raton, FL: CRC Press, 1994

95 McKeigue PM, Shah B, Marmott MG. Relation of central obesity and insulin resistance with high diabetes prevalence and cardiovascular risk in South Asians. *Lancet* 1991; **337**: 382–6

96 Sobal J, Stunkard AJ. Socio-economic status and obesity: a review of the literature. *Psychol Bull* 1989; **105**: 260–75

97 Rossner S. Cessation of smoking and body weight increases. *Acta Med Scand* 1986; **219**: 1–2

98 Prentice AM, Jebb SA. Obesity in Britain: Gluttony or sloth. *BMJ* 1995; **311**: 437–9

99 Law CM, Barker DJP, Osmond C, Fall CHD, Simmonds SJ. Early growth and abdominal fatness in adult life. *J Epidemiol Community Health* 1992; **46**: 184–6

100 Prokopec M, Bellisle F. Adiposity in Czech children followed from 1 month of age to adulthood: analysis of individual BMI patterns. *Ann Hum Biol* 1993; **20**: 517–25

101 Must A, Jacques PF, Dallal GE, Bajema CJ, Dietz WH. Long-term morbidity and mortality of overweight adolescents; a follow-up of the Harvard Growth study of 1922 to 1935. *N Engl J Med* 1992; **327**: 1350–5

102 Williamson DF, Madans J, Pamuk E, Flegal JS, Kendrick JS, Serdula MK. A prospective study of childbearing and 10-year weight gain in US white women 25 to 40 years of age. *Int J Obes* 1994; **18**: 561–9

103 Wing RR, Matthews KA, Kuller LH, Meilahn EN, Plantinga PL. Weight gain at the time of menopause. Arch Int Med 1991; **151**: 97–102

104 Wadden TA. Treatment of obesity by moderate and severe caloric restriction. Results of clinical research trials. *Ann Intern Med* 1993; **119**: 688–93

105 Williamson DF, Madans J, Anda RF, Kleinman JC, Giovino GA, Byers T. Smoking cessation and severity of weight gain in a national cohort. *N Engl J Med* 1991; **324**: 739–45

106 Epstein LE, Valoski AM, Vara LS, McCurley J, Wisniewski L *et al.* Effects of decreasing sedentary behaviour and increasing activity on weight change in obese children. *Health Psychol* 1995; **14**: 109–15.

107 DiGuiseppi C, Roberts I, Li L. Influence of changing travel patterns on child death rates from injury: trend analysis. *BMJ* 1997; **314**: 710–2

Obesity management by life-style strategies

Gill Cowburn*, **Melvyn Hillsdon**[†] and **Catherine R Hankey**[§]

Health Education Authority, The Churchill, Oxford, UK; [†]Health Promotion Sciences Unit, London School of Hygiene and Tropical Medicine, London, UK; [§]University Department of Human Nutrition, Glasgow Royal Infirmary, Glasgow, UK

This chapter discusses lifestyle management strategies for obesity in adults and is based on an assumption that treatment, resulting in appropriate and sustained weight loss, is of benefit to individuals. It examines dietary management strategies including the use of very low calorie diets, moderate energy restriction and individual and group approaches in commercial and non-commercial environments. It explores the role of physical activity in the treatment of obesity in particular focusing on the associated health benefits and the increasing evidence of the importance of physical activity in weight maintenance. It discusses the effect of behavioural interventions on achieving and maintaining weight loss and briefly offers suggestions for the organisation of lifestyle interventions.

This chapter deals with lifestyle management strategies for obesity in adults. It is split into three main sections dealing with interventions involving adoption of dietary management, those designed to influence exercise or physical activity behaviour and interventions which include aspects of behavioural management. It also gives suggestions for the organisation of lifestyle interventions.

This paper is based on an assumption that treatment, resulting in appropriate and sustained weight loss, is of benefit to individuals who are overweight or obese. The links between obesity and ill-health are well established[1,2] and there is growing consensus that reduction of even small amounts of weight may confer health benefits[3,4]. There remain, however, concerns about the hazards of periods of weight loss followed by weight regain[5] and some argue that the benefits of treatment of obesity have been overstated[6].

There is an abundant body of literature[6a] relating to obesity but it is difficult to draw firm conclusions about effective treatment interventions for several reasons. Firstly, published research may inform about the efficacy of interventions in the study population rather than provide evidence which is generalisable to the whole obese population[7,8]. Secondly, there is evidence that traditional methods of assessing dietary intake and level of physical activity, such as diary keeping, may be unreliable[9]. Finally, there is no consistent definition of a successful treatment, although efforts have been made to address this[3,10].

*Correspondence to:
Gill Cowburn,
Health Education
Authority, Block 10,
The Churchill,
Oxford OX3 7JL, UK*

Dietary management strategies

Research suggests that most of the benefit of weight loss is achieved when people have lost 5–10 kg[3], which is equivalent to 35,000–70,000 kcal. As the loss of 1 kg represents 7000 kcal, weight management should aim for a maximum weight loss of 0.5–1 kg/week. Reducing weight more quickly than this increases the physiological strain following acute energy deficit and the risks of weight regain. Brownell and Wadden[4] suggest that the likelihood of an obese person achieving sufficient weight loss to reach their ideal body weight is remote, and physical and psychological benefits of moderate weight loss are apparent much earlier after only moderate weight loss. Estimates have been made that 95% of those slimming on their own fail to lose 95% of their overweight[11] although it is possible that many such slimmers already have an acceptable body mass index (BMI), and would have only gained cosmetic, rather than health, benefits from weight reduction.

By convention, those with BMI below 25 kg/m² are not considered overweight[12,13] and an appropriate approach to support these people is advice for weight maintenance. There are some circumstances, however, where weight reduction would be recommended[14] when BMI is between 21–24 kg/m². This would include individuals with non-insulin dependent diabetes (NIDDM) or where the genetic risk of NIDDM is high.

The need for weight loss, rather than just avoiding further weight gain, is increased when the BMI is above 30 kg/m² or the BMI is 25–30 kg/m² in the presence of a central fat distribution or with secondary complications such as NIDDM, hyperlipidaemia and hypertension.

Very low calorie diets (VLCD) in weight management

Weight loss with VLCD Very low calorie diets are 'complete diet' regimens, usually liquid drinks but which may include a daily meal based on solid food. Energy provision is less than 3300 kJ/800 kcal/day[12–14]. The use of VLCD was extensively reviewed by the US Task Force on the Prevention and Treatment of Obesity[13] which concluded that supervision by a physician and the selection of patients with a BMI greater than 30 kg/m² should provide appropriate and adequate safeguards to their use. The most frequent complication in the use of VLCD was cholelithiasis, the extent of which was described by Yang[13]. In his study of 100 subjects undertaking VLCD therapy for 16 weeks, 10% of subjects developed clinically recognisable symptoms of gallstones.

Mean weight losses with VLCD range from 1.5–2.5 kg/week, so that use over 12–16 weeks will produce close to a 20 kg weight loss. This compares with a weight loss of 0.5–0.6 kg/week using a less extreme 5000 kJ/1200 kcal approach, leading to a weight loss of 6–8 kg over the same time. The speed of weight loss tends to slow with VLCD as basal metabolic rate is suppressed by a mean of 15%[17].

The acceptability of VLCD regimens was investigated by Wadden *et al.*[18], where a VLCD was compared with a similar energy provision achieved using food. No differences in actual weight loss were seen between the two groups although the 'food' based diet was rated as being more acceptable by subjects. In practice, also, individuals tend to revert to their usual life-style and use the VLCDs only intermittently, which may be a judgement against the acceptability of VLCD.

VLCD regimens have been used in many short term weight reducing studies with considerably fewer examining their long term use[19]. Foster *et al.*[20] used either an intermittent 500 kJ/1200 kcal regimen, or a constant 5000 kJ/1200 kcal daily regimen for 20 weeks in two over-weight patient groups with weight losses of 9.5 and 8 kg, respectively. Using estimates of energy requirements, an expected weight loss would be close to 27.5 and 22 kg, respectively. The shortfall between calculated and actual weight loss suggests poor adherence to the programme.

Maintenance of weight loss after VLCD   Maintenance of weight loss continues to be a major concern with all approaches to weight management but, in particular to the VLCD, which attempt to induce the greatest calorific deficit in comparison with actual energy require-ments. Flynn and Walsh[21] enrolled overweight, healthy subjects on a VLCD regimen for a period of 26 weeks. The weight loss achieved for 90% of subjects, after 26 weeks, was 10% body weight and this was maintained by 33% of subjects in 30 month follow-up. The initial weight loss was 21.4 kg, and maintained weight loss was 6.5 kg.

Weight maintenance with VLCD in NIDDM patients was examined by Wing *et al*[22]. There was greater weight loss with VLCD when compared with conventional hypocaloric diet (14.5 kg *versus* 10.5 kg) at 50 weeks. These differences were due to differences in weight loss after the first 12 weeks of dietary treatment. Interestingly, the authors did not consider the differences in weight losses important enough to justify the use of a VLCD regimen in preference to a conventional dietary regimen.

Longer study periods show extended periods of weight stability or maintenance, rather than an increase in total weight loss. Accrued weight losses are comparable for the use of VLCD whatever the duration of the study. Caprio Shovic *et al.*[23] examined a 16 week VLCD programme whose recruits were subject to rigorous follow up. Weight loss was 15 kg (15% body weight) for men and 15 kg (9% body weight) for women, but 18 months after this programme was complete, there was no remaining weight loss for the two-thirds of subjects for whom data were available.

Osterman *et al.*[24] tested a structured programme which combined a VLCD (12 weeks/2500 kJ/600 kcal) with a period of relaxing the dietary regimen to 5000 kJ/1200 kcal for 6 weeks and finally a period of weight maintenance on a Step 1 national cholesterol education programme for a further 7 weeks. At 25 weeks, weight loss was 25 kg, suggesting improved adherence on this structured programme. Long term weight maintenance after the programme, however, was not evaluated.

Safer *et al.*[25] reviewed the long term maintenance of weight loss after VLCD and concluded that, after 12 months, 75% of dieters regain most of their lost weight. After 2 years, this figure rises to 85–90%[26].

Moderate energy restriction for weight loss

The use of a food based dietary plan or regimen which is usually 5000 kJ/1200 kcal per day or above, is an established approach to weight reduction. These programmes are most often administered on an individual subject and therapist basis. They may or may not include advice to increase physical activity. Svedsen *et al.*[27] investigated the effect of moderate weight loss using a 5000 kJ/1200 kcal diet which was accompanied by increased physical activity in one group of overweight women, and diet alone in another. Both groups had maintained respectable weight losses (of 10.6 kg in exercisers and 6.6 kg in non exercisers) at 9 months post intervention.

As attempts to gauge energy requirements from dietetic assessments usually give unreasonable results[28], the value of prescribing an energy intake derived from predictions of metabolic rate based on age, sex and weight has been proposed. Lean and James[28] advocate that dietary prescriptions which incorporate a daily energy deficit of 2000 kJ/ 500 kcal below estimated energy requirements, in the place of a blanket approach where all-comers would be given 5000 kJ/1200 kcal, are adopted. The same diet for everyone, in practice offers a lower energy prescription in relation to estimated energy requirements to those most overweight, compared to their less overweight counterparts. Frost *et al.*[29] compared this energy deficit approach to a conventional 5000 kJ/ 1200 kcal diet. Patients attending a dietetic weight management clinic were randomised either to a 5000 kJ/1200 kcal regimen or an individually calculated diet prescription with a daily energy deficit of 2000 kJ/500 kcal. The results showed the value of a more lenient prescription, which was rewarded with greater weight losses in the individually prescribed group when compared with the standard advice group. Another recent study[30,31] in a healthy but overweight group of volunteers, using a daily 600 kcal deficit approach, achieved similar weight losses of 5%, though an identical study group of overweight volunteers with established angina achieved poorer weight loss (4%) which may have been influenced by the poor physical activity level within this group.

Group versus individual approaches to weight management

The value of a group approach has been described[32] as offering a cost effective environment for effective weight management[33]. Whilst the group environment is undoubtedly unsuitable for some shy or reluctant socialisers, for those agreeable to this approach it allows additional harnessing of structure and support, not accessible to the subject undergoing individual, one-to-one, dietary counselling.

The Harrow slimming club uses an approach similar to that used by commercial organisations. However, it is run under the National Health Service, by State Registered Dietitians and although clients are fee paying, it is non profit making[34]. The ten session weekly programme consists of individual weighing, dietary advice and education. The dietary approach is identical for all-comers and is based on a 5000 kJ/ 1200 kcal dietary prescription. An audit of the club showed a weight loss of 5.4 kg for those who attended eight of the ten sessions. This was reduced to 3.8 kg in those attending around seven sessions[27]. There are no long term data examining the effectiveness of the club, though it is almost alone in being both non-commercial and having its effectiveness evaluated. Another similar approach to weight management is the Finnish Primary Health Care programme[35]. This study used a 1200 kcal diet group, and a control group who were followed up, but offered no advice. After the 6 week weight reduction course, which included behavioural advice, follow-up meetings were arranged at monthly and twice monthly intervals. Men reduced their weight by 10.9 kg at 1 year, and women 5.4 kg over the same time period. After a lengthy 7 year follow-up, men had maintained weight losses of 8.7 kg and women 3.5 kg.

Advantages for group therapy in comparison with conventional therapy in newly diagnosed diabetic patients have been described[36] though in established overweight diabetic patients no advantage was found by Blonk et al[37]. The impressive results of Jeffery et al.[38] favoured group therapy.

Commercial slimming organisations

There is little published information about the effectiveness of commercial slimming groups, though non-commercially run groups are reported in the literature. The commercial groups themselves suggest that their treatments, together with a measure of financial commitment, are effective[19]. However, attrition remains a major problem[39] and an early study suggested the compliance half-life for commercial slimming varies from 10–50 weeks[40]. Ashwell and Garrow showed a 9.3 kg weight loss (11.3% of starting weight) over 6 months[41]. However, these results are based on self reported body weights from subjects who had been approached and willing to provide this information. Those subjects who were unwilling may represent study failures.

A non-commercial slimming group approach was taken by Cousins *et al*[42]. This study evaluated a family based slimming programme against a diet sheet, or dietary advice given on an individual basis in overweight subjects. The individuals allocated not to receive group treatment in the diet sheet and individual advice groups lost 1–2 kg over the 1 year study period. The whole family slimming group achieved losses of 4–5 kg. The American Take Off Pounds Sensibly (TOPS) programme reported a similar degree of success[43]. Garb and Stunkard[40] found that weight loss was related to the length of attendance, and to the initial degree of overweight.

Lay helpers

Brownell and Jeffery[44] compared the use of lay helpers in a slimming group with a comparable group guided by qualified health professionals. No differences were found in the success of weight loss between the two groups. Nuutinen and Knip[45] described the use of counsellors (in this case trained children) to act as leaders in children's slimming sessions. The success of counselling and group therapy in weight control appears to depend not only on the depth of knowledge of a particular person, but on their approach to others and their success in gaining group approval and trust.

Summary of dietary management interventions

The current dietary management of overweight and obesity succeeds in achieving moderate weight losses, which are increasingly being acknowledged as leading to recognised health benefits. The use of VLCD regimens are proven to achieve good weight losses over the short term, though scant evidence exists to support their value for weight loss maintenance.

The moderate energy deficit approach has been shown to be effective in achieving weight losses around 5 kg over a 12 week programme. It may be that the use of a moderate energy deficit will favour the maintenance of weight loss, with the losses having been achieved gradually.

The value of group approaches to weight loss have been established in clients amenable to a more sociable programme. Group treatments harness structure and support from others, in addition to the educational opportunities presented by the programme. Commercial slimming organisations and organisations of lay helpers may offer similar advantages with some clients finding the financial outlay an additional incentive. Assessment of the weight loss results of the commercial slimming organisations may offer possibilities in maximising treatment effectiveness.

Physical activity interventions and weight management

A report by the US Surgeon General on physical activity and health highlighted the significant health benefits which are associated with regular physical activity[46]. They include: (i) lowered all cause mortality; (ii) decreased risk of cardiovascular disease mortality; (iii) prevention or delayed development of hypertension; (iv) reduced blood pressure in those with hypertension; (v) decreased risk of colon cancer; (vi) decreased risk of developing non-insulin dependent diabetes; and (vii) relief from symptoms of depression and anxiety.

Yet, despite these benefits, a large proportion of the population do not engage in sufficient amounts of physical activity to obtain them. In England, it is estimated that 70% of the population are insufficiently active[47]. The 1994 Health Survey of England[48] reported a significant inverse association between physical activity and BMI in both men and women. Men who engaged in at least three occasions of moderate or vigorous exercise per week had a mean BMI 0.79 kg/m^2 (95% CI, −1.06, 0.52) lower than men doing no physical activity, whereas in women the difference was 1.14 kg/m^2 (95% CI, −1.14, 0.8). Other cross sectional studies have shown similar results. A population based survey in the US reported the prevalence of physical inactivity (defined as no participation in leisure time physical activity during the preceding month) in overweight people (BMI ⩾ 27.8 kg/m^2 for men and ⩾ 27.3 kg/m^2 for women). 41% (95% CI, 38.8, 42.2) of overweight women and 33% (95% CI, 31.6, 34.4) of overweight men were classified as inactive, compared to 30.1% (95% CI, 30.1, 31.3) and 26.5% (95% CI, 25.9,

27.1), respectively, in the whole population. Men and women who were obese (BMI $\geqslant 31.1 \, \mathrm{kg/m^2}$ for men and $\geqslant 32.3 \, \mathrm{kg/m^2}$ for women) were even more likely to be inactive, 38% (95% CI, 35.6, 40.4) and 46% (95% CI, 43.8, 48.2), respectively[49].

Another American study reported on 10 year weight gain among 3515 men and 5810 women. Cross sectional analyses of both surveys revealed that the relative risk of significant weight gain (> 13 kg) during the 10 year period for subjects engaging in low levels of recreational activity at both surveys, was 2.3 (95% CI, 0.9, 5.8) in men and 7.1 (95% CI, 2.2, 23.3) in women[50].

Cross sectional data show a strong association between physical inactivity and overweight. However, one of the limitations of cross sectional data is that causal inferences cannot be made so it is unclear whether low levels of physical activity are a cause or consequence of weight gain.

Prospective studies of physical inactivity and obesity have shown less consistent results than cross sectional studies. The study by Williamson *et al.*[50] found no relationship between baseline levels of physical activity and subsequent weight gain among either men or women. Another prospective study found that both leisure time physical activity and work activity predicted changes in body weight over time in women but not in men[51]. A study of the determinants of weight gain in adult men and women from Finland found that the prevalence of obesity was inversely associated with physical activity: 12,669 adults were examined on two occasions with a median follow up period of 5.7 years. The relative risk (adjusted for potential confounders) of weight gain (5 kg or more) in 5 years for those who exercised less than once per week compared to those who exercised three or more times per week, was 1.9 (95% CI, 1.5, 2.3) for men and 1.6 (95% CI, 1.2, 2.2) for women[52].

A study among 22,076 male health professionals determined the relative risk of becoming overweight during 2 years of follow-up. The relative risk (adjusted for potential confounders) for becoming overweight was 0.81 (95% CI, 0.65, 1.01) in the most active compared with the least active men[53].

In summary, there appears to be an inverse relationship between physical activity and obesity, although the direction of the relationship is less clear. Prospective studies provide provisional evidence for suggesting that a population increase in physical activity could help prevent an increased prevalence of obesity over time.

Physical activity in the treatment of obesity

When physical activity or exercise alone is used in the treatment of obesity, weight losses are modest and average 2–3 kg[54]. However, evidence does exist that exercise alone can produce much larger reductions in weight when it is of sufficient frequency, intensity and duration[55]. There appears to be a dose–response relationship between level of exercise and degree of weight lost[55]. One study which compared dieting versus exercise on weight loss and lipoproteins, in a 1 year randomised controlled trial, found that both intervention groups lost significant weight compared to controls. Dieters lost an average of 7.2 kg after 12 months compared to exercisers who lost an average of 4.0 kg ($P < 0.01$)[56].

A combination of diet and exercise generally produces greater weight losses than diet alone[57–60], although this is not always so[61]. One study which randomised dieters to exercise or no exercise found that the exercise group lost an average of 10.8 kg during the 12 week intervention period compared to 8.1 kg ($P < 0.05$) in the diet only group. Perhaps more importantly, subjects in the exercise group adhered to the prescribed diet better than the no exercise group[62].

One of the most consistent findings in studies of exercise in the treatment of obesity is the effect on weight maintenance. During one study, subjects who had participated in a 12 month randomised controlled trial of the effects of weight loss through exercise or diet were randomly assigned to either a weight maintenance treatment or an assessment only control group[63]. The maintenance strategy involved regular mailed information packs and telephone contact. The amount of initial weight lost that was regained in intervention compared with control groups was different for exercisers compared to dieters. Although dieters had lost more weight than exercisers after 12 months, dieters regained 42% of weight lost compared to exercisers who only regained 17.4% of weight lost ($P < 0.01$). Similar findings occurred in the study by Skender et al.[60], who also followed subjects for 2 years. After 12 months, dieters had lost an average of 6.8 kg, exercisers 2.9 kg and the diet plus exercise group 8.9 kg ($P=0.9$). At 2 years, dieters had reached a weight 0.9 kg above baseline, the diet plus exercise group 2.2 kg below baseline and the exercise only group 2.7 kg below baseline, only 0.2 kg greater than that at 1 year. This meant that the total weight change at 2 years was greatest in the exercise only group. Due to relatively small numbers, differences did not reach statistical significance ($P=0.36$), but group by time interaction was observed ($P < 0.001$), suggesting that the longer the follow-up the greater the weight regained.

Eighteen month follow-up data of a study which randomly assigned subjects to different dietary interventions and to exercise or no exercise, showed no difference in weight regained between the different dietary regimens. However, comparisons between exercisers and non exercisers showed a significant difference in weight loss maintained ($P < 0.001$). All non exercise groups regained nearly all of the weight lost during the 8 week treatment period compared to the exercisers who maintained most of the weight lost[58].

Two of the few studies to follow subjects who had taken part in commercial weight loss programmes both found that maintenance of weight lost was associated with frequency of exercise[64,65].

The results of these follow-up studies suggest that, although exercise is associated with smaller weight losses than dieting in the short term, it is associated better weight maintenance post intervention. A 'U' shaped curve best describes the change of body weight over time achieved through dieting alone. Therefore, it is reasonable to conclude that subjects who successfully achieve and maintain a lower body weight are likely to be exercisers. However, the existing data do not allow us to determine whether exercise is anything more than a marker for good dietary compliance, as suggested by Racette *et al.* [62].

A meta-analysis of the effect of exercise, with or without dieting on the body composition of overweight adults, aimed to determine if physical activity conserved fat free mass (FFM), often lowered during dieting. The studies reviewed were divided into the following four categories: (i) subjects on a weight maintenance diet assigned to exercise or no exercise; (ii) subjects on a weight maintenance diet and exercise or more restricted diet without exercise; (iii) exercising and non exercising subjects both on energy restricting diets not less than 1000 kcal/day; and (iv) exercising and non exercising subjects both on energy restricting diets less than 1000 kcal/day.

Results of the analyses suggest that exercise, and in particular resistance training exercise, results in an increase in FFM in subjects on an adequate diet. In addition, for any given weight loss, the loss of FFM will be less in exercising versus non exercising subjects. The findings of this meta-analysis are important as FFM is the best predictor of resting metabolic rate which in turn is the largest contributor to total daily energy expenditure. Any reduction in FFM is likely to lead to a reduction in total daily energy expenditure, making weight loss more difficult[66].

Potential mechanisms linking exercise with weight maintenance include: (i) enhanced resting metabolic rate; (ii) preservation of lean tissue during weight loss; (iii) increased total daily energy expenditure; and (iv) increase in post exercise oxygen consumption. For a complete review of these mechanisms, readers are referred to Hill *et al.*[67].

How much exercise is required?

The US Surgeon General's report[46] on physical activity and health recommends that:

Activity leading to an increase in daily expenditure of approximately 150 kilocalories/day (equivalent to about 1,000 kilocalories/week) is associated with substantial health benefits and that the activity does not need to be vigorous to achieve benefit.

This amount of physical activity can be met in a number of different ways. The most frequently cited example is walking briskly for 30 min/day on most, preferably all, days of the week. This more moderate message is encouraging for obese subjects who are unlikely to tolerate the more traditional message of 20 min of vigorous activity on at least 3 days/week. However, the new, more moderate, message is not intended to replace the older recommendation. Additional health and fitness benefits are associated with more vigorous intensity activity.

Although these recommendations were not specifically designed for obese people, they have been included in the US Department of Health and Human Services Dietary Guidelines for weight maintenance[68]. The American College of Sports Medicine has recommended that weight loss programmes include a programme of exercise that promotes a daily caloric expenditure of 300 kcal or more[69].

Recent research has suggested that intermittent bouts of exercise accumulated during the course of the day may have fitness benefits similar to one longer bout of exercise. However, it is not known whether this holds true for the health outcomes associated with continuous exercise[46]. Nevertheless, this approach to physical activity promotion may be easier to achieve for obese subjects. In a study of overweight women, subjects were randomly assigned to either a short-bout (SB) exercise group or a long-bout (LB) exercise group. All subjects were encouraged to exercise 5 days/week and recommended the same caloric intake. The LB group performed one bout of exercise per day, whereas the SB group performed multiple bouts of 10 min. Both groups were encouraged to start with 20 min of exercise per day building up to 40 min. At 20 weeks, the SB group exercised on a greater number of days ($P < 0.05$) and for a greater duration than the LB group ($P=0.08$). The amount of weight lost was similar in both groups[70].

Can physical activity be increased?

A systematic review of physical activity promotion strategies[71] found some evidence that physical activity can be increased in previously sedentary subjects. Only 11 randomised controlled trials were identified that met the inclusion criteria, none from the UK and none which particularly targeted obese subjects. The review concluded that interventions that encouraged walking and did not require attendance at a facility are more likely to lead to sustainable increases in overall physical activity. The review also found that regular follow-up by a professional improves the proportion of people able to maintain increased levels of physical activity. The finding that walking is associated with better compliance is consistent with the new recommendations for health.

Summary of physical activity interventions

Research consistently shows an inverse relationship between energy expenditure from physical activity and lower body weight. It also seems likely that low physical activity contributes to the development of obesity and its maintenance. Obese subjects who engage in a programme of regular physical activity achieve modest reductions in weight. Although such reductions are less than might be achieved through dietary approaches, they are more likely to maintained post intervention. Exercise combined with caloric restriction appears to achieve the greatest reductions in weight as well as enhancing fat loss and minimising FFM loss.

Programmes which emphasise frequent, moderate intensity exercise, such as brisk walking, are more likely to lead to sustainable increases in physical activity.

In addition to the benefits of a lower weight, physically active obese subjects are at a lower risk of all cause and cardiovascular mortality, compared to the sedentary obese independent of changes in weight.

Behavioural management

Behavioural interventions use strategies in addition to provision of diet and physical activity information to facilitate change. Programmes encourage individuals to become aware of their eating and physical activity behaviours and focus on changing the environmental factors which control their behaviour, specifically the cues that precede the behaviour and the reinforcers that come after the behaviour and lead to its recurrence[72].

Behavioural treatments and weight loss

Behaviour modification was first used in obesity treatment in the 1960s, when early treatments focused on self-monitoring of food intake and associated behavioural patterns as well as stimulus control techniques, avoiding triggers that produce problem behaviours[73]. Newer programmes are more comprehensive, being longer in duration, putting more emphasis on nutrition education, and increasing physical activity; they also include social support, skills-building, cognitive-behavioural strategies and relapse[73-75]. The latter programmes appear to be more successful at achieving weight loss[44], which may be positively associated with treatment duration, hours of therapist contact and therapist experience[76] and intensity of programme[72].

Behavioural treatments are complex and identifying the important elements within programmes remains a challenge. Cameron et al.[77] evaluated a correspondence weight control programme assessing the impact of different programme elements, namely printed lessons, weekly homework, interim weigh-ins and participation deposits. Women in all treatment groups, except lessons only, showed a greater BMI reduction than untreated controls at the end of treatment. At 1 year follow-up, women receiving printed lessons and weekly homework had a greater mean weight loss (3.93 ± 4.88 kg) when compared to lessons only group (0.34 ± 4.45 kg).

The role of the spouse in behavioural treatment of obesity was studied by Rosenthal et al.[78], where the effect of full husband involvement, partial husband involvement or no husband involvement was examined. Women with full or partial husband involvement showed greater weight loss (4.67 kg and 4.94 kg, respectively) compared to women with no husband involvement (3.22 kg) post-treatment ($P < 0.001$), but no significant differences were demonstrated at 3 year follow-up. Pearce et al.[79] examined spouse involvement in a small study, using a restricted calorie intake in addition to behavioural treatment, with mixed results.

Cognitive strategies which include cognitive restructuring, self-instructional training and rational-emotive therapy have been included in behavioural programs[75]. These strategies attempt to help people to improve their thinking and thereby improve their behaviours and emotions[80]. Cognitive strategies may be used in conjunction with behavioural treatments, for example Perri[81] used this approach in a study to assess the effect of lengthening duration of treatment. A similar intervention was delivered to each group, with one treatment group subject to 20 weekly sessions and the other group subject to extended 40 weekly sessions. The extended treatment group achieved a significantly greater weight loss ($P < 0.05$) post treatment (-13.64 ± 9.00 kg) compared to the shorter treatment group (-6.41 ± 5.99 kg) and an overall statistically significant with time effect ($P < 0.05$). The significantly greater weight loss for the extended treatment group was maintained at 72 week follow-up.

Wadden et al.[18] assigned women to one of three treatments: VLCD alone; behaviour therapy alone; or a combination of VLCD and behaviour therapy. Those in the combined treatment group lost significantly greater weight ($P < 0.03$) at the end of treatment (-16.8 ± 1.2 kg) when compared to the other two groups (-13.1 ± 1.0 kg and -13.0 ± 1.4 kg, respectively). At 1 year follow-up, the combined treatment group showed significantly greater weight losses ($P < 0.04$) than those in the diet alone group (-10.6 ± 1.6 kg and -4.7 ± 1.5 kg, respectively). Differences among conditions were significant ($P < 0.05$), with both behaviourally treated groups superior to VLCD alone group. The majority of subjects in all three treatment groups, however, had returned to their pretreatment weight 5 years after treatment.

Wing et al.[82] compared behavioural treatment alone and in combination with written menu plans and grocery lists; written menu plans, grocery lists and a partially subsidised food box; and written menu plans, grocery lists and a free food box. After the 6 month intervention, those in the behaviour treatment only group had achieved significantly less weight loss ($P < 0.003$) than the other groups (8.0 ± 6.2 kg compared with 12.0 ± 7.2 kg, 11.7 ± 5.4 kg and 11.4 ± 6.5 kg, respectively) which was maintained ($P < 0.02$), despite some regain across all groups, at 1 year follow-up.

Maintaining weight loss with behavioural treatments

In reviewing weight loss maintenance following behavioural treatment programmes, Brownell and Jeffery[44] and Wing[72] conclude that weight loss appears to be maintained in the first year following treatment, followed by a gradual regain. Booster sessions, monetary contracts, ongoing support groups and mail and telephone follow-up have been evaluated, with support for the effectiveness of these approaches being unclear[83].

Perri et al.[84] compared the effect of behavioural therapy, relapse prevention training and post-treatment contact by mail and phone on maintenance of weight loss against several variants including no further follow-up and a non-behavioural therapy control. All groups achieved weight loss post treatment but only those receiving behaviour therapy plus relapse prevention training plus post-treatment contact by mail and phone maintained their post-treatment weight loss at 1 year follow-up.

Perri et al.[85] continued to explore client–therapist contact where subjects were assigned to one of three groups following a standard 20 weeks of behavioural treatment: a peer self-help group maintenance programme; therapist contact maintenance programme; or no maintenance programme. At 7 month follow-up, the therapist contact group had achieved greater weight loss (-11.54 kg) than either the peer self-help or control groups (-9.31 kg and -7.82 kg, respectively) but this difference was not maintained at 18 months follow-up.

Perri *et al.* extended their work in this area[83] by assigning subjects to five different groups comparing behaviour therapy alone with a four variants of behaviour therapy plus post-treatment therapist contact maintenance programme; post-treatment therapist contact plus a social influence maintenance programme; post-treatment therapist contact plus aerobic exercise maintenance programme; or post-treatment therapist contact plus social influence programme plus aerobic exercise programme. At 18 months follow-up, all four conditions combining behaviour therapy with post-treatment maintenance gave greater weight loss than behaviour therapy alone.

The use of daily weight charts as part of a behavioural treatment was tested by Fujimoto *et al*[86]. A significant between group difference ($P < 0.05$) was shown at 2 year follow-up, with those assigned to the behaviour therapy plus daily weight chart group achieving a mean weight change of -14.8 kg compared with those receiving behaviour therapy alone achieving a mean weight change of -8.8 kg.

Summary of behavioural interventions

Behavioural treatments appear to achieve weight loss successfully, especially as part of a comprehensive intervention, lasting for at least 16 weeks, which includes building social support, cognitive behavioural strategies and skills building in addition to emphasis on nutrition education and increasing physical activity.

Maintaining weight loss, at least to 1 year post intervention, seems to be associated with increasing length and intensity of programme, relapse prevention training and with maintenance of therapist contact.

Outline for treatment organisation

The wider context within which people live must be considered in order to gain insight into the challenges of obesity lifestyle treatments. Whilst individuals may undoubtedly change their behaviour to lose and maintain body weight, especially by undertaking comprehensive treatment programmes supported by appropriately trained 'therapists', activity is required to create a more supportive environment in which successful change may be achieved. Recommendations for a population approach to help address the problem of obesity have been suggested[87].

Lifestyle treatment strategies should be aimed at those individuals most likely to benefit, for example those with a BMI over $30 \, \text{kg/m}^2$ or those with a BMI $25-30 \, \text{kg/m}^2$ with additional risk factors such as central adiposity, NIDDM or hypertension and hyperlipidaemia. Individuals should be offered treatment options[4,44,88] and treatment should include an assessment of readiness to change[89–91]. It should also address, for example, self-efficacy, an individual's confidence in his/her ability to make changes, which has been applied to predict intention to diet, weight loss and retention of loss by several investigators. Individuals who had initial high weight-loss self-efficacy were usually most successful in achieving their goals[75]. Treatment programmes should be more comprehensive, emphasising behaviour modification, physical activity, nutrition education, cognitive-change strategies and social support. They should aim to provide longer interventions with a greater emphasis on maintenance and relapse prevention[73,92] and, perhaps, focus upon goals other than weight loss, including a cessation of weight gain or improved ability to cope in the absence of weight loss as well as looking for improvements in lifestyle, health risk factors, body image and self-esteem[75].

References

1   Health Education Authority. *Obesity in Primary Health Care: A Literature Review*. Health Education Authority: London, 1995

2   Garrow JS. *Obesity and Overweight*. Health Education Authority: London, 1991

3   Goldstein DJ. Beneficial health effects of moderate weight loss. *Int J Obes* 1992; **16**: 397–415

4   Brownell KD, Wadden TA. The heterogeneity of obesity: fitting treatments to individuals. *Behav Ther* 1991; **22**: 153–77

5   Anonymous. *National Task Force on the Prevention and Treatment of Obesity. Weight Cycling*. JAMA 1994; **272**: 1196–202

6   Wooley SC, Garner DM. Obesity treatment: the high cost of false hope. *J Am Diet Assoc* 1991; **91**: 1248–51

6a   NHS Centre for Reviews and Dissemination, University of York. *Systematic Review of Intervention in the Treatment and Prevention of Obesity*. 1997; In press

7   Fitzgibbon ML, Stolley MR, Kirschenbaum DS. Obese people who seek treatment have different characteristics than those who do not seek treatment. *Health Psychol* 1993; **12**: 342–5

8   Brownell KD. Whether obesity should be treated. *Health Psychol* 1993; **12**: 339–41

9   Lichtman SW, Pisarska K, Berman ER *et al*. Discrepancy between self-reported and actual caloric intake and exercise in obese subjects. *N Engl J Med* 1992; **327**: 1893–8

10   Atkinson RL. Proposed standards for judging the success of the treatment of obesity. *Ann Intern Med* 1992; **119**: 677–80

11   Perri MG, Nezu AM, Viegner BJ. *Improving the Long Term Management of Obesity*. New York: Wiley Bioscience, 1992

12   Royal College of Physicians. *Obesity, a Report of the Royal College of Physicians*. London: Royal College of Physicians, 1983

13   National Task Force on the Prevention and Treatment of Obesity. *Very low calorie diets.* *JAMA* 1993; **270**: 967–74

14   Colditz GA, Willett WC, Rotnitzky A, Manson JE. Weight gain as a risk factor for clinical diabetes in women. *Ann Intern Med* 1995; **122**: 481–6

15   Department of Health. *Dietary Reference Values, Report 41.* London: HMSO, 1991

16   Yang H, Petersen GM, Roth MP, Schoenfield LJ, Marks JW. Risk factors for gallstone formation during rapid loss of weight. *Dig Dis Sci* 1992; **37**: 912–8

17   Garrow JS, Webster JD. Effects on weight and metabolic rate of obese women on a 3–4 mJ (800 kcal) diet. *Lancet* 1989; **i**: 1429–31

18   Wadden TA, Sternberg JA, Letizia KA, Stunkard AJ, Foster GD. Treatment of obesity by very low calorie diet, behavior therapy and their combination, a five year perspective. *Int J Obes* 1989; **13 (Suppl)**: 39–46

19   Hymans FN, Sempos E, Saltsman N. Evidence for the success of caloric restriction in weight loss and control. *Ann Intern Med* 1993; **119** 681–7

20   Foster GD, Wadden TA, Peterson FJ. A controlled comparison of three very low calorie diets: effects on weight, body composition, and symptoms. *Am J Clin Nutr* 1992; **55**: 811–7

21   Flynn TJ, Walsh MF. Thirty month evaluation of a popular very-low calorie diet programme. *Arch Fam Med* 1993; **2**: 1042–7

22   Wing RR, Greeno CG. Behavioral and psychosocial aspects of obesity and its treatment. *Ballieres Clin Endocrinol Metab* 1994; **8**: 689–703

23   Caprio Shovic A, Adams S, Dubitzky J, Anacker M. Effectiveness and dropout rate of a very low calorie diet program. *J Am Diet Assoc* 1993; **93**: 583–4

24   Osterman J, Lin T, Howard R, Brown KA, Horning CA. Serum cholesterol profiles during treatment of obese outpatients with a very low calorie diet. Effect of initial cholesterol levels. *Int J Obes* 1992; **16**: 49–58

25   Safer DJ. Diet behavior modification and exercise: a review of obesity treatment from a long term perspective. *South Med J* 1991; **84**: 1470–3

26   Sikand G, Kando A, Foreyt JP. Two year follow-up with a very low calorie diet and exercise training. *J Am Diet Assoc* 1988; **88**: 487–8

27   Svedsen OL, Hassager C, Christiansen C. Six months' follow-up on exercise added to a short term diet in overweight postmenopausal women—effects on body composition, resting metabolic rate, cardiovascular risk factors and bone. *Int J Obes* 1994; **18**: 692–8

28   Lean MEJ, James WPT. Prescription of a diabetic diets for the 1980s. *Lancet* 1986; **i**: 723–5

29   Frost G, Masters K, King C *et al.* A new method of energy prescription to improve weight loss. *J Hum Nutr Diet* 1991; **4**: 369–74

30   Hankey CR, Rumley A, Lowe GDO, Lean MEJ. Weight loss improves established indices of ischaemic heart disease risk. *Proc Nutr Soc* 1995; **54**: 94A

31   Hankey CR, Wallace AM, Lean MEJ. Plasma lipids, dehydroepiandrosterone sulphate and insulin concentrations in elderly overweight angina patients, and effect of weight loss. *Int J Obes* 1996; In press

32   Lean MEJ, Anderson AS. Clinical strategies for obesity management. *Diabetic Med* 1988; **5**: 515–8

33   Bitzen PO, Melander A, Schersten B, Svensson M. Efficacy of dietary regulation in primary health care patients with hyperglycaemia detected by screening. *Diabetic Med* 1988; **5**: 634–9

34   Bush A, Webster J, Chalmers G *et al.* The Harrow Slimming Club: report on 1090 enrolments in 50 courses, 1977–1986. *J Hum Nutr Diet* 1988; **1**: 429–36

35   Hakala P, Karvatti RL, Ronnemaa T. Group versus individual weight reduction in the treatment of severe obesity—a five year follow-up study. *Int J Obes* 1993; **17**: 97–102

36   Heller SR, Clarke P, Daly H *et al.* Group education for obese patients with type 2 diabetes: greater success at less cost. *Diabetic Med* 1988; **5**: 552–6

37   Blonk MC, Jacobs MAJM, Biesheuvel EHE, Weda-Manak WL, Heine RJ. Influences of weight loss in type 2 diabetic patients: little long term benefit from group behaviour therapy and exercise training. *Diabetic Med* 1994; **11** 449–57

38   Jeffery RW, Gerber WM, Rosenthal BS, Lindquist RA. Monetary contracts in weight control: effectiveness of group and individual contracts of varying size. *J Consult Clin Psychol* 1983; **51**: 242–8

39 Volkamar FR, Stunkard AJ, Woolston J, Bailey JF. High attrition rates in commercial weight reduction programmes. *Arch Intern Med* 1981; **141**: 426–8

40 Garb JR, Stunkard AJ. Effectiveness of a self help group in obesity control: a further assessment. *Arch Intern Med* 1974; **134**: 716–20

41 Ashwell MA, Garrow JS. A survey of three slimming and weight control organisations in the UK. *Nutrition* 1975; **29**: 347–56

42 Cousins JH, Rubovits DS, Dunn JK, Reeves RS, Ramirez AG, Foreyt JP. Family versus individually orientated intervention for weight loss in Mexican American women. *Public Health Rep* 1992; **107**: 549-55

43 Kahn HS, Williamson DF. Is race associated with weight change in US adults after adjustment for income, education and marital factors. *Am J Clin Nutr* 1991; **53**: 1566S–70S

44 Brownell KD, Jeffery RW. Improving the long term weight loss. Pushing the limits of treatment. *Behav Ther* 1987; **18**: 353–74

45 Nuutinen O, Food Sci L, Knip M. Weight loss, body composition and risk factors for cardiovascular disease in young children: long term effects of two treatment strategies. *J Am Coll Nutr* 1992; **11**: 707–14

46 US Department of Health and Human Services. *Physical Activity and Health: A Report of the Surgeon General*. Atlanta, GA: US Department of Health and Human Services, Centers for Disease Control and Prevention, National Center for Chronic Disease Prevention and Health Promotion, 1996

47 *Allied Dunbar National Fitness Survey. Main Findings*. London: Sports Council and Health Education Authority, 1992: 46

48 *Health Survey for England 1994*. London: HMSO, 1995: 282

49 Office of Surveillance and Analysis, and Division of Nutrition and Physical Activity, National Center for Chronic Disease Prevention and Health Promotion, Centers for Disease Control. Prevalence of physical inactivity during leisure time among overweight persons — behavioral risk factor surveillance system, 1994. *Morb Mortal Wkly Rep* 1996; **45**: 185–8

50 Williamson DF, Madans J, Anda RF, Kleinman JC, Kahn HS, Byers T. Recreational activity and ten-year weight change in a US national cohort. *Int J Obes* 1993; **17**: 279–86

51 Klesges RC, Klesges LM, Haddock CK, Eck LH. A longitudinal analysis of the impact of dietary intake and physical activity on weight change in adults. *Am J Clin Nutr* 1992; **55**: 818–22

52 Rissanen AM, Heliovaara M, Knekt P, Reunanen A, Aromaa A. Determinants of weight gain and overweight in adult Finns. *Eur J Clin Nutr* 1991; **45**: 419–30

53 Ching PLYH, Willet WC, Rimm EB, Colditz GA, Gortmaker SL, Stampfer MJ. Activity level and risk of overweight in male health professionals. *Am J Public Health* 1996; **86**: 25–30

54 King AC, Tribble DL. The role of exercise in weight regulation in nonathletes. *Sports Med* 1991; **11**: 331–49

55 Gwinup G. Effect of exercise alone on the weight of obese women. *Arch Intern Med* 1975; **135**: 676–80

56 Wood PD, Stefanick ML, Dreon DM *et al*. Changes in plasma lipids and lipoproteins in overweight men during weight loss through dieting as compared with exercise. *N Engl J Med* 1988; **319**: 1173–9

57 Pavlou KN, Whatley JE, Jannace PW *et al*. Physical activity as a supplement to a weight loss dietary regimen. *Am J Clin Nutr* 1989; **49**: 1110–4

58 Pavlou KN, Krey S, Steffee WP. Exercise as an adjunct to weight loss and maintenance in moderately obese subjects. *Am J Clin Nutr* 1989; **49**: 1115–23

59 Kempen KPG, Saris WH, Westerterp KR. Energy balance during an 8-week energy-restricted diet with and without exercise in obese women. *Am J Clin Nutr* 1995; **62**: 722–9

60 Skender ML, Goodrick K, Del Junco DJ *et al*. Comparison of 2-year weight loss trends in behavioral treatments of obesity: diet, exercise and combination interventions. *J Am Diet Assoc* 1996; **96**: 342–6

61 Grilo CM. Physical activity and obesity. *Biomed Pharmacother* 1994; **48**: 127–36

62 Racette SB, Schoeller DA, Kushner RF, Neil KM. Exercise enhances dietary compliance during moderate energy restriction in obese women. *Am J Clin Nutr* 1995; **62**: 345–9

63 King AC, Frey-Hewitt B, Dreon DM, Wood PD. Diet vs exercise in weight maintenance: The effects of minimal intervention strategies on long term outcomes in men. *Arch Intern Med* 1989; **149**: 2741–6

64 Grodstein F, Levine R, Troy L, Spencer T, Colditz GA, Stampfer MJ. Three year follow-up of participants in a commercial weight loss program. *Arch Intern Med* 1996; **156**: 1302–6

65 Holden JH, Darga LL, Olson SM, Stettner DC, Ardito EA, Lucas CP. Long term follow-up of patients attending a combination very low calorie diet and behaviour therapy weight loss programme. *Int J Obes* 1992; **16**: 605–13

66 Garrow JS, Summerbell CD. Meta-analysis: effect of exercise, with or without dieting, on the body composition of overweight subjects. *Eur J Clin Nutr* 1995; **49**: 1–10

67 Hill JO, Drougas HJ, Peters JC. Physical activity, fitness and moderate obesity. In: Bouchard C, Shephard RJ, Stephens T (eds) *Physical Activity, Fitness and Health: International Proceedings and Consensus Statement 1992*. Champaign: Human Kinetics, 1994; 684–91

68 US Department of Agriculture, US Department of Health and Human Services. *Nutrition and your Health: Dietary Guidelines for Americans*. 4th edn. Washington DC: US Department of Agriculture, Home and Garden Bulletin No. 232, 1995

69 American College of Sports Medicine. *ACSM's Guidelines for Exercise Testing and Prescription* 5th edn. Baltimore: Williams and Wilkins, 1995

70 Jakicic JM, Wing RR, Butler BA, Robertson RJ. Prescribing exercise in multiple bouts versus one continuous bout: effects on adherence, cardiorespiratory fitness and weight loss in overweight women. *Int J Obes* 1995; **19**: 892–901

71 Hillsdon M, Thorogood M. A systematic review of physical activity promotion strategies. *Br J Sports Med* 1996; **30**: 84–9

72 Wing R. Behavioral treatment of severe obesity. *Am J Clin Nutr* 1992; **55**: 545S–51S

73 Foreyt JP. Issues in the assessment and treatment of obesity. *J Consult Clin Psychol* 1987; **55**: 677–84

74 Wilson MA. Southwestern Internal Medicine Conference: treatment of obesity. *Am J Med Sci* 1990; **299**: 62–8

75 Parham E. Nutrition education research in weight management among adults. *J Nutr Ed* 1993; **25**: 258–68

76 Bennett GA. Behavior therapy for obesity: a quantitative review of the effects of selected treatment characteristics on outcome. *Behav Ther* 1986; **17**: 554–62

77 Cameron R, MacDonald MA, Schlegel RP *et al*. Towards the development of self-help health behavior change programs: weight loss by correspondence. *Can J Public Health* 1990; **81**: 275–9

78 Rosenthal B, Allen G, Winter C. Husband involvement in the behavioral treatment of overweight women: initial effects and long term follow-up. *Int J Obes* 1980; **4**: 165–75

79 Pearce JW, LeBow MD, Orchard J. Role of spouse involvement in the behavioral treatment of overweight women. *J Consult Clin Psychol* 1981; **49**: 236–44

80 Ellis A, Abrams M, Denglegi L. *The Art and Science of Rational Eating*. New Jersey: Barricade Books, 1992

81 Perri MG, Nezu AM, Patti ET, McCann KL. Effect of length of treatment on weight loss. *J Consult Clin Psychol* 1989; **57**: 450–2

82 Wing R, Jeffery R, Burton L, Thorson C, Sperber Nissinoff K, Baxter J. Food provision v structured meal plans in the behavioral treatment of obesity. *Int J Obes* 1996; **20**: 56–62

83 Perri MG, McAllister DA, Gange JJ, Jordan RC, McAdoo WG, Nezu AM. Effects of four maintenance programs on the long term management of obesity. *J Consult Clin Psychol* 1988; **56**: 529–34

84 Perri MG, Shapiro RM, Ludwig WW, Twentyman CT, McAdoo WG. Maintenance strategies for the treatment of obesity: an evaluation of relapse prevention training and post-treatment contact by mail and telephone. *J Consult Clin Psychol* 1984; **52**: 404–13

85 Perri MG, McAdoo WG, McAllister DA *et al*. Effects of peer support and therapist contact on long term weight loss. *J Consult Clin Psychol* 1987; **55**: 615–7

86 Fujimoto K, Sakata T, Etou H *et al*. Charting of daily weight pattern reinforces maintenance of weight reduction in moderately obese patients. *Am J Med Sci* 1992; **303**: 145–50

87 Department of Health. *Obesity: Reversing the Increasing Problem of Obesity in England*. A report from the Nutrition and Physical Activity Task Forces. London: Department of Health, 1995

88 Committee to Develop Criteria for Evaluating the Outcomes of Approaches to Prevent and Treat Obesity. Summary: weighing the options: criteria for evaluating weight management programs. *J Am Diet Assoc* 1995; **95**: 97–105

89 Prochaska JO, Velicer WF, Rossi JS *et al*. Stages of change and decisional balance for twelve problem behaviours. *Health Psychol* 1994; 13, 1, 39-46

90 O'Connell D, Velicer WF. A decisional balance measure and the stages of change model for weight loss. *Int J Addict* 1988; **23**: 729–50

91 Rollnick S. Behaviour change in practice: targeting individuals. *Int J Obes* 1996; **20** (**Suppl. 1**): 22–6

92 Perri MG, Sears SF, Clark JE. Strategies for improving maintenance of weight loss: towards a continuous care model of obesity management. *Diabetes Care* 1993; **16**: 200–9

Present and future pharmacological approaches

Nick Finer

Centre for Obesity Research, Luton and Dunstable Hospital, Luton, UK

There is evidence that drugs altering food intake such as dexfenfluramine, sibutramine and orlistat have useful therapeutic effects, with an acceptable side effect profile. 'Thermogenic' drugs, such as ephedrine and caffeine, are also effective, but less well tolerated and may, in any case, work by producing anorexia. The state of drug treatment for obesity now is similar to the early days of anti-hypertensive treatment in the 1960s when reserpine, ganglion blockers and non-selective adrenergic blocker were all that was available. There is considerable reason for optimism that the next 10 years will bring better treatments for the obese.

Concepts of pharmacological management

Previous chapters have highlighted the health risks and diseases that result from obesity. In such circumstances one would expect pharmacological treatment to be welcomed as a useful adjunct to other treatment modalities. Yet, for many years, drug treatment of obesity has been regarded as a hallmark of poor clinical practice. Until recently the *British National Formulary* stated[1]: 'drugs can play only a limited role and should never be used as the sole element of treatment; their effects tend to be disappointing'. In 1995, the Medicines Control Agency proposed to restrict the use of 'medicinal products which act upon the central nervous system so as to suppress the appetite' to those with a new definition of 'severe obesity based up a definition of a body mass index of greater or equal to 35 kg/m^2', because 'the products are recognised as having the potential for creating dependency and have a range of severe side effects'. A recent paper auditing prescribing performance of general practitioners, marked the prescription of appetite suppressants as poorly as prescribing more than 60% of drugs non-generically[2].

Why are anti-obesity drugs held in disrepute? The reasons for this appear to arise, in part, because many fail to recognise the importance of obesity both as a disease, and as a cause of disease. In part there has also been a long-standing mis-evaluation of the pharmacology of anti-obesity drugs. The medical establishment has been slow to accept the health implications of obesity and has shown many of the same prejudices as

Correspondence to:
Dr Nick Finer,
Centre for Obesity
Research, The Luton and
Dunstable NHS Trust,
Lewsey Road, Luton,
Bedfordshire LU4 0DZ,
UK

British Medical Bulletin 1997;**53** (No. 2): 409–432

the public in stigmatising obese patients. Doctors are more likely regard obese people as 'weak-willed . . . and awkward' than lean counterparts[3,4]. With this background, in which obesity is the patient's 'own fault', it is easy to conclude that the obese are not 'worthy of drug treatment' and thus undervalue drug intervention[5]. Accepting obesity as disease, and recognising the limitations of non-drug treatments such as diet, exercise and behaviour modification, inevitably leads to the conclusion that effective drug treatments are needed. There is nothing unusual about such a conclusion, since a similar one has existed concerning many other chronic diseases, such as hypertension and diabetes mellitus. Both these require pharmacological intervention for long-term control. The spectrum of body weight from serious disease (obesity), medical risk (overweight), healthy (normal), to underweight (thin), opens it to the pressures of fashion and desire for cosmetic change (slimming). The use of drugs for 'treating' normal or thin people is widespread and clearly undermines the value of the same drugs when used to treat obesity. The pejorative and dismissive collective noun of slimming pills reflects such a prejudice against this therapeutic area.

It is encouraging that the recent greater understanding of the physiological basis, and the health implications of obesity, together with recognition of the limitations of existing non-drug treatment, is gradually dispelling this era of negativity. A number of consensus statements — from bodies such as the North American Association for the Study of Obesity (NAASO)[6] and the UK Association for the Study of Obesity (ASO)[7] — have recognised the need and logic of drug treatment. In Scotland, the Scottish Intercollegiate Guidelines Network (SIGN)[8] has highlighted the need for drug treatment 'in selected patients'. Official and regulatory bodies are also increasingly adopting more realistic attitudes to drug treatment. The UK Medicines Commission[9] recently concluded in its review of anorectic medication, that 'the criteria applied to the use of appetite suppressants should be similar to those applied to the treatment of other chronic relapsing disorders'. In the US, the Food and Drugs Administration (FDA) has issued guidance concerning the standards of clinical efficacy they wish to see for registering new anti-obesity treatments (Table 1). The FDA has recently licensed or approved two centrally acting anorectic drugs, dexfenfluramine and sibutramine. These changes have lead to an explosion of interest and research by the pharmaceutical industry, such that a large number of anti-obesity drugs are in development.

A traditional methodology of drug development applied to obesity might hypothesise that a single molecule, with a well defined mechanism of action at the appropriate molecular or biochemical target, would reverse the causes of excessive weight gain and restore a healthy body weight. The inherent complexity of body weight regulation makes such a

Table 1 FDA guidance on the development of drugs for treating obesity

- Encourage development of new drugs that will be efficacious, safe, for specific aetiology
- Foster development for long–term or indefinite use
- Demonstrate benefit greater than with diet, exercise, behaviour modification alone
- Weight loss on drug treatment at 12 months exceeds placebo by at least 5% of baseline weight
- Significant improvement in co–morbid conditions and/or quality of life
- Exhibit safety commensurate with efficacy and projected duration of use

goal unrealistic, and it seems that a drug to 'cure' obesity is much less likely than a cure for diabetes mellitus or hypertension. In obesity treatment, drugs should be seen not as 'magic bullets', but as an adjunct to behavioural change. Treatment should aim to control or ameliorate the disease, relieve symptoms and enhance life quality and expectancy. To achieve these goals, a drug must at least induce, accelerate or help maintain weight loss; preferably it will do all three. Since patients present with a wide range in the severity of their obesity, an ideal anti-obesity drug would produce dose-related weight loss with a wide dose-response range. There has, however, been a common tendency to misinterpret the effects of anti-obesity drugs. Figure 1 shows schematic graphs of the fall in weight with an anti-obesity drug, and the fall in blood glucose with an anti-diabetic medication. Table 2 shows how misinterpretation of these outcomes can bias against recognising the worth of an anti-obesity drug. Thus there is no requirement for an anti-hypertensive drug to lower blood-pressure progressively and indefinitely, nor for it to be effective after it is discontinued. Asking whether it is better that an obese person takes a drug and stays 10% lighter, or not take the drug and remain 10% heavier is a simple way of demonstrating the logic of drug treatment. At present, there is a reliance of surrogate measures of benefit (weight loss, reduction in risk factors such as blood-pressure, dyslipaemia, etc.) rather than hard outcome measures, such as mortality and morbidity. Evidence does exist, however, for the benefits of modest weight loss insufficient to normalise body weight[10–13]. However, in the quest for hard measures of therapeutic efficacy, softer measures of benefit, such as improved quality of life, must not be discounted or ignored. As for any treatment to be given long-term, there is a need for long duration studies of efficacy and safety, and this does pose considerable practical difficulties both in designing controlled trials, and in funding them[14].

The principles of treating obesity with drugs, and the onus to prescribe wisely, therefore do not differ from any other disease. Drugs must be shown to be safe and effective with a high benefit to risk ratio[15]. At an individual level, treatment efficacy must be established and monitored. with the patient being seen regularly. Since the goal of treatment is

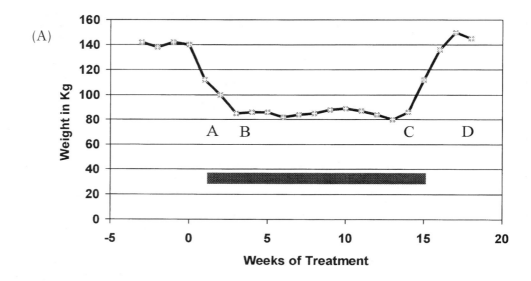

(A)

(B)

Fig. 1 Schematic illustration of effect of anti-obesity medication on body weight (A) and anti-diabetic medication on blood glucose (B). The shaded bar shows the duration of drug treatment. Differing interpretations of drug effects highlight bias against anti-obesity medications (see Table 2).

weight loss maintenance, treatment will need to be continued long-term, although periods of drug withdrawal are likely to be helpful in establishing that treatment really does need to be continued.

In developing drug treatments for obesity, it would be rational to look for drugs that act on those components of physiology or pathophysiology that are perturbed. Epidemiological evidence suggests that it is, in population terms, the combination of low activity levels with a ready food supply, high in fat, that has lead to the rapid increase in

Table 2   Interpretation of patterns of weight loss and blood–glucose lowering (Fig 1A,B)

	Anti–obesity drug Usual misinterpretation	Anti–obesity drug Correct interpretation	Anti–diabetic drug Usual interpretation
A	Drug started unnecessarily because patient failed to alter life-style. Patient doesn't need or deserve drug treatment	Drug treatment needed to reduce risks of obesity	Drug treatment needed because life-style changes inadequate to correct disease and unsafe to leave blood glucose at this level
B	Failure of drug to normalise body weight means drug didn't work	Worthwhile effect of drug, despite failure to normalise weight	Worthwhile effect of drug, despite failure to normalise blood glucose
C	Plateau shows that drug tolerance has developed	Plateau shows continued efficacy of drug. Level of weight loss maintenance may or may not be sufficient to justify long-term drug continuation	Plateau shows continued efficacy of drug. Desirable that blood glucose does not fall lower and lower
D	Regain of weight after drug withdrawal shows that the drug did not work	Regain of weight shows that drug was still effective, and that long-term treatment is necessary	Regain of elevated blood glucose shows that drug treatment must be continued

prevalence[16]. However, at the individual level, the causes for obesity, or for that matter leanness, are less clear. This lack of knowledge means that, to some extent, drug treatment remains empirical and any drug that reduces energy intake, increases energy expenditure or alters energy storage could be of potential benefit. Table 3 classifies anti-obesity drugs and lists some of those available or under development.

Evaluating drug therapy

The bedrock of assessing anti-obesity drugs, randomised controlled trials, does not differ from any other area of medical intervention. Trials must be designed to allow clinically meaningful questions to be answered, and be of sufficient statistical power to give valid positive or negative answers. The disease of obesity, as a disease, usually presents with specific clinical complications such as diabetes mellitus, ischaemic heart disease, stroke, cancer, etc. Measures of body weight, therefore, act only as a surrogate for the real end-points of clinical interest. Surrogate end-points are useful because they allow studies to be conducted more cheaply and easily. For example, compared to measuring body weight, measuring body fat is time consuming, expensive and may involve exposing the subject to ionising radiation. Other advantages of surrogate measures include the use of smaller sample sizes and the ability to measure outcomes more quickly (e.g. body weight loss rather than infarction rates). However, it is always important to be aware that the quality of a surrogate measure diminishes the further it is from the endpoint of interest. Thus a study measuring

Table 3 Classification of anti–obesity drugs by main mode of action. Drugs licensed or in Phase III development are listed in bold. Those of questionable efficacy are in brackets

Energy intake	Energy storage	Energy Output
Brain	Fat	Brain
Behaviour modifier	*Decreased lipid storage*	*Stimulant*
serotoninergic	?GH	**noradrenergic**
dexfenfluramine	? leptin	
sibutramine	insulin sensitisers	
Anorexia	Ro 23-7637	Muscle + BAT
serotoninergic	Troglitazone	*Thermogenic*
dexfenfluramine		β_3 agonists
sibutramine		**Thyroid hormones**
noradrenergic	*Increased lipid oxidation*	**Ephedrine**
Phentermine	α_2 antagonists	**Caffeine**
Mazindol	(Yohimbine)	**Aspirin**
Diethylpropion		?serotoninergic
(PPA)		(Dinitrophenol)
sibutramine		?noradrenergic
peptidergic		
NPY antagonists		
? leptin		
enterostatin		
GI Tract		
Delayed gastric emptying		
CCK promoters		
Butabindide		
chlorocitric acid		
Relay to brain		
CCK promoters		
Nausea/aversive		
Malabsorption		
orlistat		

weight loss alone could fail to recognise that a drug could produce weight loss through adverse events such as sedation and nausea, rather than anorexia or increased energy expenditure; a fall in body weight due to loss of lean tissue could be harmful rather than beneficial.

Obesity presents particular problems for clinical trials. Although the disease is easy to diagnose, it is heterogeneous and methods for defining different phenotypes are poor. Subjects recruited tend to be women who represent only half of the obese population at risk. There is a long lag time for the development of obesity to its complications, and weight loss remains poorly validated as a surrogate measure for events such as ischaemic heart disease or cancer. Weight loss maintenance over years rather months is the desired aim of any treatment but, in clinical trials, there is often a high drop-out rate (about 40% in most studies) and often poor or partial compliance. The reasons for the high attrition rates in trials are not clear, but relate in part to a patient's own perception of obesity as a cosmetic and life-style problem rather than a disease.

Although there is evidence to suggest that a loss of 10% from baseline will give medical benefit[10,13], and reduce the costs of health care of the co-morbid conditions[6], we do not really know how much weight loss is optimal. Since visceral fat loss provides the greatest risk to health, measures of regional fat loss may be more important than total weight loss when treatment benefits are evaluated.

The US FDA has given guidance on standards of evidence necessary to achieve registration for a new compound (Table 1). The philosophy is that drugs should be developed for long-term or indefinite use, and demonstrate benefit greater than can be achieved with diet, exercise and behaviour modification alone. Anti-obesity drugs must exhibit safety commensurate with their efficacy and projected duration of use. Safety and toxicology studies will precede initial short term studies (12–24 weeks) to establish dosage and efficacy. Double-blind studies of 1 year duration are needed, and 2 years in special situations. Efficacy would be judged as loss of 5% of body weight with improvement in co-morbid diseases or risk factors, or 10% if there is no co-morbidity. Since anti-obesity drugs can be expected to be used widely and for long periods of treatment, Phase IV, post-marketing surveillance studies, must be designed and implemented. The issuing of such guidance in the US, achieved by a NAASO task force and the FDA and Federal Trade Commission, has had a galvanising effect on industry. Pharmaceutical companies and researchers, in the US, now know the standard of evidence needed to achieve new drug registration.

Drugs that predominantly reduce food or energy intake

In order to maintain the obese state, energy intake must be sustained sufficiently high to meet the increased metabolic demands of the large body mass. Control of food intake is complex, and has evolved to favour increased consumption; only weak mechanisms (mainly cognitive) exist to protect against the high fat, high palatability foods and low energy life-style of developed societies[17]. Early drugs to be used for treating obesity were amphetamine or amphetamine derivatives. A meta-analysis of 200 controlled trials included nearly 10,000 patients in trials of 4–20 weeks duration. In 90% of trials, active drug was superior to placebo with weight loss on average 0.23 kg/week greater[18]. Scoville noted that although drugs 'do not provide complete cures, ... [there] is no reason to reject them out of hand; partial success is clearly better than failure'. Despite this, his report has often be misinterpreted as suggesting anorectics were ineffective. The more recent development of serotoninergic drugs, such as fenfluramine and dexfenfluramine, without stimulant properties, has gone some way to renew interest in appetite suppressants.

Amphetamines

The discovery of ephedrine from the Chinese plant *Ephedra sinica*, led to the synthesis of the amphetamines in 1933[19]. Initially used as stimulants, it soon became apparent that these drugs also suppressed appetite and food intake[20], useful not only for the obese but also for logistical military advantage in World War II. The potent abuse and addictive potential of these drugs makes them unsuitable for use.

Phenylethylamines and other catecholaminergic 'stimulant' drugs

These were developed to preserve the anorectic actions of amphetamines, but have weaker stimulant activity than amphetamine and no addictive potential. In rodents these drugs increase sympathetic activity and stimulate thermogenesis[21], but not in man where the anti-obesity action is mediated through central nervous system anorexia. Diethylpropion (amfepramone) has less stimulant activity than amphetamine[22] and reduces subjective ratings of hunger. The risks of abuse appear to be small[23,24]. A trial of 200 patients receiving diethylpropion for 24 weeks showed weight loss of between 6.6 and 11.3 kg, although only 18% of patients completed the trial[25]. Another, smaller, trial over 23 weeks showed weight loss of 11.7 kg with the active drug compared to 2.4 kg in those given placebo[26]. A strategy of intermittent treatment (1 month on, 1 month off) proved as effective as continuous treatment[27]. Despite these findings, the drug's stimulant properties made it poorly tolerated by patients (and their prescribers), and in a recent climate of disapproval of stimulant anorectic drugs, has been voluntarily withdrawn from the UK. Phentermine has similar properties and in one trial showed about 8 kg more weight loss than placebo over 36 weeks, regardless of whether the drug was given continuously or intermittently[28]. Mazindol (an imidazoisoindole) has a longer half-life than the phenylethylamines (33–55 h) and also is superior to placebo at producing weight loss[29]. The pitfall of trying to evaluate an anorectic drug in combination with a highly restricted diet was shown in one study in which Mazindol or placebo was giving together with a 260 kcal/day semi-synthetic diet[30]. Clearly with such a restricted diet, there was little or no room to measure any additional efficacy from the anorectic drug; nor was dietary compliance enhanced by Mazindol which had to be withdrawn in 6/25 patients because of side effects. This group of drugs is little used as sole agent, but may be usefully combined with other drugs (see later).

Phenylpropanolamine

This racemic mixture or norephedrine esters is available over the counter in the US and is a component of many 'cold cures'. These drugs release noradrenaline throughout the body, which can act at a wide variety of adrenergic receptors. The predominant action is to stimulate hypothalamic adrenoreceptors so to reduce appetite, rather than increase thermogenesis[31]. Phenylpropanolamine has a low abuse potential and has no adverse effects on blood pressure at recommended doses[29,32]. It is superior to placebo at producing weight loss, but the difference in weight is modest, 0.7–1.8 kg over 4–12 weeks[33]. It is widely used as an OTC preparation in the US.

Serotoninergic drugs

Fenfluramine was synthesised in the 1960s by the introduction of a trifluoromethyl group into the phenyethylamine ring[19]. Although for many years it was classified as a catecholaminergic drug, it was clear from animal and human clinical studies that the drug had no stimulant activity, and that its mechanism of action differed from the other phenylethylamines[34]. While amphetamines release dopamine and noradrenaline within the lateral hypothalamus, fenfluramine acted as a releaser and re-uptake inhibitor of serotonin in presynaptic neurones terminating within the paraventricular nucleus of the hypothalamus. Serotonin anorexia differs from that caused by amphetamines; it is characterised by a decreased rate of eating and early termination of meals, rather than an inhibition of eating[35]. These anorectic effects of serotonin are mediated by $5HT_{2B}$ and $5HT_{2C}$ receptors (stimulation of $5HT_{1A}$ receptors increases food intake; stimulating $5HT_3$ receptors has no effect on food intake)[36]. A large literature on fenfluramine exists and was reviewed in 1975[37]. Fenfluramine is a mixture of two racemic compounds, l-fenfluramine and d-fenfluramine, which are metabolised to active, but pharmacologically distinct, products l-norfenfluramine and d-norfenfluramine. The d-isomer (dexfenfluramine) was found to have greater activity at reducing food intake in rats, and have a greater specificity for serotonin release and reuptake inhibition, while the l-isomer had greater dopaminergic activity[19,38].

Dexfenfluramine was developed during the 1970s, and licensed in Europe in the 1980s, and in North America in 1996. Several reviews have been published[39–41]. Tables 4 and 5 detail some of the many clinical trials of dexfenfluramine in uncomplicated obesity, and obesity associated with non-insulin dependent diabetes. Randomised controlled trials of dexfenfluramine 15 mg twice daily, with or without dietary intervention, support its efficacy at producing clinically significant weight loss superior to placebo. Longer term studies show continued efficacy for up to 1 year, the longest trial period so far reported. The International Dexfenfluramine study (INDEX)[42] included 822 patients, from 24 centres in 9 European countries. Patients were included if their body weight was 120% ideal, stable to within 3 kg over the preceding 3 months, and within 85% of their highest recorded weight. Each centre added dexfenfluramine to their usual treatment protocol (varying from formula diets, lifestyle advice or simple dietetic management). This study demonstrates important lessons on how to interpret the results of anti-obesity trials. Judged by weight loss of completing patients, the difference between active drug and placebo, while significant, appears small (Fig. 2). However, these data bias against the drug effect, because significantly more placebo-treated patients dropped out because of dissatisfaction at their lack of weight loss (84) compared to dexfen-fluramine-treated patients (49). Figure 3 presents the results on the numbers of patients achieving, arbitrary, but clinically valid weight-loss targets. Taking dexfenfluramine, approximately doubled the chances of an individual reaching more than 10% or 10 kg loss. More recent analysis of the INDEX data has allowed the prediction of long-term results from the early response to treatment[43]. A loss of 1.8 kg or more after 4 weeks of treatment positively predicted 48% of patients who achieved a loss of 10% or more at 1 year. Failure to lose 1.8 kg after 1 month, had a negative predictive value of 90%. A weight loss of 10% or more after 4 months predicted 84% of those achieving a similar weight loss at 1 year; failure to lose 10% weight by month four predicted 90% of those failing to achieve this target at 1 year. These figures have been incorporated into the prescribing indications in North America.

Unwanted effects of dexfenfluramine are relatively minor and short-lived[40,44]. A review of 1159 patients treated with dexfenfluramine and 1138 with placebo over 3 months showed diarrhoea (17.5% vs 7.3%) and dry mouth (12.5% vs 5%) to be the most common side effects[45]. Withdrawal rates from trials were similar between dexfenfluramine and placebo treated patients (6.6% and 5.2%). Pulmonary hypertension (PPH), a potentially fatal condition, has been associated with the fenfluramines[46]. A large case control study, the IPPHS[47], collected all cases of PPH (95) from 220 hospitals over 25 months to investigate the association with anorectic medication. Obesity itself, and systemic

Table 4 Summary of trial data of dexfenfluramine in treating uncomplicated obesity

	Trial size	BMI/IBW	Duration/diet/ exercise	Outcome	Comments
Finer et al.1985[96]	89 A and P	BMI ∼ 32	12 weeks	A: − 4.1 kg (4.8% init bw)	Hospital and GP subjects
			30% decrease energy	P: 0 kg	RCT
Enzi et al. 1988[97]	64 A and P	BMI ∼ 32	12 weeks	A: − 8.1 kg (9.8% init bw)	
			Hypocaloric diet	P: − 3.5 kg (3.8% init bw)	
Finer et al. 1988[98]	29 Active	IBW ∼ 147%	24 weeks 30% decrease energy	− 7.0 kg (8.3% init bw)	Open label continuation after 12 week RCT
Finer et al. 1992[99]	47 A and P	BMI ∼ 44	24 weeks 70% caloric needs assessed from RMR	A: − 6.0 kg P: +3.0 kg	Patients had already lost 13.9 kg on a VLCD
Noble 1990[100]	42 A and P	BMI ∼ 37 kg	24 weeks 1200–1500 kcal/ day	A: − 6.2 kg P: − 2.6 kg	
Guy-Grand et al. 1989[42]	822 A and P	IBW ∼ 158%	52 weeks	A: − 9.8 kg (10.3% init bw)	Higher completion in A group
			Variable	P: − 7.2 kg (7.2% init bw)	
Mathus- Vliegen et al. 1992[101]	75 A and P	BMI ∼ 38	12 weeks 50% or 1000 kcal/day reduction	A: − 10.7 kg P: − 8.0 kg	
Pfohl et al.1994 [102]	48 A and P	IBW ∼ 156%	52 weeks 1200(M)–1500 (F) kcal/day	A: − 10.9 kg (11.2% init bw) P: − 9.6 kg (9.1% init bw)	2 years after drug withdrawal, A group +1.5 kg, P − 2.1 kg. INDEX subgroup
Drent et al. 1995[103]	112 A and P	BMI ∼ 32	9 weeks no dietary advice	A: − 3.1 kg. ↓ fat, CHO, energy; ↓ standing BP P: +0.2 kg	Included if waist- hip ratio > 1.0 in M, 0.8 in F, > 5 snacks daily totalling > 500 kcal or 25% total intake
O'Connor et al. 1995[104]	60 A and P	BMI ∼ 35	26 weeks Lifestyle programme 1500(M)–1200(F) kcal/day	A: − 9.74 kg P: − 4.9 kg	5 months after drug withdrawal, drug effect negated with wt loss 6.0 and 6.2 kg
Lucas et al. 1995[105]	337 A and P	BMI ∼ 34	12 weeks	A: − 5.8 kg	No change in Hamilton D ratings
			Variable dietary advice	P: − 1.9 kg	

Abbreviations: A, active treatment, P placebo. IBW, ideal body weight. BMI, body mass index. init bw, initial body weight. M, male, F, female. CHO, carbohydrate. BP, blood pressure. RCT, randomised controlled trial. VLCD, very low calorie diet.

hypertension increased the risk of PPH (1.9- and 2.1-fold, respectively), and exposure to any centrally anorectic medication also increased the risk of PPH (10.1-fold for recent, and 2.4-fold for past exposure). Treatment for more than 3 months further increased the odds ratio to 23.1. However, PPH is extremely rare (1–2 cases/million) and so the

Table 5 Summary of trial data for treating obese NIDDM patients

Obese NIDDM	Trial size	BMI/IBW	Duration/diet/ exercise	Outcome	Comments
Tauber Lassen et al 1990[106]	35 A and P	BMI ∼ 34	52 weeks 1200–1440 kcal/day	A: — 5.7 kg P: — 2.7 kg	
Stewart et al. 1993[107]	60 A and P	BMI ∼ 35	12 weeks	A: — 3.7 kg P: +0.4 kg	Significant fall in fasting BG and glycated in A group
Willey et al. 1992[108]	34 A and P	BMI ∼ 34	12 weeks	A: — 3.8 kg P: — 0.6 kg	Significant fall in glycated Hb and fructosamine in A group
Manning et al.1995[109]	205		12 + 40 weeks	DF: — 2.8 kg Clinic visits: — 1.2 kg Behaviour program: — 1.8 Home visits: — 1.1 kg Control: +1.2 kg	Patients assigned to dexfenfluramine for 3 months, regular clinic, group behavioural programme, home visits, or no intervention

Abbreviations: A, active treatment, P placebo. IBW, ideal body weight. BMI, body mass index. init bw, initial body weight. M, male, F, female. CHO, carbohydrate. BP, blood pressure. RCT, randomised controlled trial. VLCD, very low calorie diet.

absolute risk is very low—about 28 cases/million person-years of exposure. This incidence is similar to the risks of death from penicillin anaphylaxis, or oral contraceptive-induced thromboembolism and myocardial infarction[48].

There has been considerable interest in the potential of fenfluramines to increase energy expenditure. Results in man have been contradictory, perhaps influenced by the conditions of study[49]. Breum et al. studied obese women over 24 h in a direct calorimeter and failed to show any effect of dexfenfluramine on energy expenditure[50]. On the other hand, Schutz and colleagues studied normal weight men with indirect calorimetry using a ventilated hood, and showed a higher rise in metabolic rate after dexfenfluramine compared to placebo (6% vs 2%), and a greater thermic response to eating a standardised a meal (22% vs 16%)[51]. A second study in obese women showed that dexfenfluramine increased post-absorptive energy expenditure by 2.5%, by extrapolation equivalent to an extra 40 kcal/24 h[49]. A thermogenic effect could thus explain how weight loss is maintained despite the increase in energy intake after 6 months treatment in long-term trials such as INDEX.

Other serotonin agonist drugs evaluated as anti-obesity agents include the selective serotonin re-uptake inhibitors such as fluoxetine[29], fluvoxamine[52] and sertraline[53]. Normally used to treat depression, these

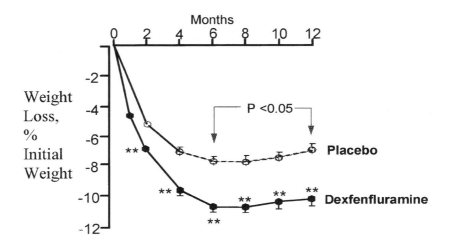

Fig. 2 Mean weight loss ($\pm$ SEM) in completers on dexfenfluramine (n=256) and placebo (n=227). Weight loss was significantly (P < 0.001) greater in dexfenfluramine to placebo patients from 2–12 months. There was a significant (P < 0.05) regain in weight between 6 and 12 months in the placebo group. Redrawn from Guy-Grand et al.[42]

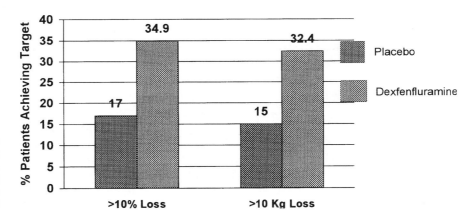

Fig. 3 INDEX study data shown on an intention to treat basis, with weight at last visit carried forward. Redrawn from Guy-Grand et al.[42]

drugs were recognised as producing weight loss rather than weight gain usually associated with tricyclic antidepressants. The doses of fluoxetine required to produce weight loss, however, are substantially higher than those used to treat depression[54]. At these doses, the drug may no longer be acting solely on serotonin neurones, but probably has effect on dopaminergic neurones also[36]. A large trial compared continued treatment with Fluoxetine 20 mg, 60 mg daily or placebo for efficacy in weight loss maintenance in 317 patients who had already lost > 3.6 kg with 8 weeks of single-blind fluoxetine treatment[55]. Within 8 weeks of the maintenance phase, all three groups of patients started to regain weight and continued to do so up to 48 weeks, findings confirmed by others[56,57].

Sibutramine

This drug, which is expected to receive US approval for registration in 1997, is a serotonin and noradrenaline re-uptake inhibitor (SNRI). It was developed initially as an anti-depressant and bears a close structural resemblance to viloxazine. Devoid of anti-depressant activity, it decreases food intake through β_1 and $5HT_{2A/2C}$ receptor agonist activity, and is thought to enhance metabolic rate through stimulation of peripheral β_3 receptors. Dose response trials over 12 weeks have shown weight loss of 5.2–6.9 kg at a dose of 10 mg daily, and 7.6 kg at 20 mg daily (manufacturer's data on file). In a 24 week, double-blind, dose finding, controlled trial in 173 patients, 10, 15, 20 and 30 mg daily produced similar maximal loss (6.1–8.3 kg)[58]. A meta-analysis of these data suggests that the percentage of patients losing 5% of baseline body weight after 12 weeks is 19% for placebo, 49% for sibutramine 10 mg, and 55% for sibutramine 15 mg.

A 1 year trial has established long-term efficacy showing weight loss of 4.8 kg for 10 mg daily, and 6.1 kg at a 15 mg daily dose[59]. Weight loss with sibutramine (10 mg daily) has been compared to dexfenfluramine 15 mg twice daily in two studies[60]. Both studies showed a trend to greater weight loss over 12 weeks with sibutramine but this was not statistically significant. A short-term study in patients with NIDDM showed weight loss at 12 weeks of 2.4 kg compared to 0.1 kg in placebo-treated patients with a non-significant fall in glycated haemoglobin of 0.4%[61]. Adverse effects include nausea, insomnia, dry mouth, rhinitis and constipation. However, the noradrenergic effects of the drug can cause an increase in heart rate and blood pressure in some individuals, or prevent the expected fall in these parameters with weight loss. The clinical importance of these adverse effects has not yet been established.

Orlistat

Orlistat inhibits pancreatic and gastric lipases, thus decreasing ingested triglyceride hydrolysis[62]. It produces a dose-dependent reduction in dietary fat absorption, which is near maximal at a dose of 120 mg thrice daily[63]. These actions lead to weight loss in obese subjects[64]. A short-term, 12 week, study showed that together with a low fat diet, orlistat produced a dose-dependent increase in weight loss (placebo, 2.9 kg; orlistat 30 mg daily, 3.61 kg; 180 mg daily, 3.69 kg; 360 mg daily, 4.7 kg; intention-to-treat analysis)[65]. A 1 year controlled trial of orlistat 360 mg daily in 267 obese patients showed weight loss of 8.5%, compared to 5.4% for placebo-treated patients. 28% of orlistat-treated patients lost more than 10% of initial body weight compared to 17% of the placebo group, judged in an intention-to-treat analysis[66]. Adverse effects of orlistat are predominantly related to gastro-intestinal effects due to fat malabsorption. These include loose or liquid stools, faecal urgency and oil discharge, and can be associated with fat-soluble vitamin absorption. Since the consumption of a high fat meal will inevitably lead to severe gastro-intestinal symptoms, it is possible that some of the weight loss with orlistat treatment is due an 'antabuse effect' enforcing behaviour change. Registration was applied for by the manufacturer, Hoffman-La Roche, in 1997.

Drugs that predominantly increase energy expenditure

Interventions that increase exercise and activity are valuable components of any weight control programme and correlate strongly with success at weight loss maintenance[67]. It is often difficult, however, for the severely obese patient to be physically active. Changing this area of behaviour may be as much as a problem for patients as a voluntary change in eating habits. For the past 20 years, there has been a concerted search for drug treatments that might safely increase metabolic rate in obese patients, and dissipate excessive energy stores as heat. The term thermogenic drugs has been coined to describe this mode of action. Since many obese patients have already, or are at risk from, ischaemic heart disease and hypertension, it would be essential that a thermogenic drug would have only minimal, if any, effect on raising heart rate, cardiac output, myocardial oxygen consumption, or blood pressure.

Dinitrophenol

Dinitrophenol was the first synthetic thermogenic drug used to treat obesity. Its thermogenic action was noticed by munitions workers at the turn of the century, and shown to result from the uncoupling of oxidative phosphorylation from ATP formation. Unfortunately, during the 1930s when it came into clinical use, there were a number of deaths from multi-system side effects, and the drug was rapidly withdrawn.

Thyroid hormones

Since the turn of the century, thyroid hormones (thyroxine and tri-iodothyronine) have been known to increase metabolic rate and thermogenesis. Patients with spontaneous overactivity of thyroid hormone production (thyrotoxicosis) have increased resting metabolic rate, often lose weight (in the face of increased appetite and food intake), and report increased sensations of heat and sweating. The mechanisms by which thyroid hormones (and in particular tri-iodothyronine) increase metabolic rate are not fully understood but involve uncoupling of oxidative phosphorylation, increasing Na^+/K^+-ATPase activity and increasing mitochondrial metabolism[68]. Since thyroid hormone-induced increases in respiration are tightly coupled to the utilisation of high energy phosphorus compounds (e.g. ATP), it seems unlikely that these biochemical processes account for the thyroid hormones' thermogenic actions; increasing the actions of catecholamines, or increasing turnover of glycogen and protein, seem more likely explanations.

In clinical practice, thyroxine and tri-iodothyronine are not useful for treatment. While they increase metabolic rate, they cause tachycardia and may provoke dysrhythmias or myocardial infarction, and are also associated with accelerated protein (fat free mass) loss. Even when used to treat hypothyroidism, weight changes are minimal[69,70]. Research into thyroid hormone analogues is in progress, and one animal study showed the possibility of combining thyroid hormone with a β-blocker[71].

Ephedrine and xanthines

Phenylpropanolamines, such as ephedrine, and xanthine derivatives, such as caffeine, increase metabolic rate. The amount of caffeine contained in two cups of coffee, 100 mg, will raise metabolic rate by about 4%, but the effect is short-lived, and may be followed by a period of reduced energy expenditure. Erikson, a Danish general practitioner, noted that asthmatic patients prescribed these drugs, involuntarily lost weight[72]. Ephedrine and caffeine appear to act synergistically, and the combination is marketed in Denmark as the Elsinore pill[72]. The actions of ephedrine are mediated through sympathetically-released noradrenaline, which could act at β_3 receptors (on brown adipose tissue), β_2 receptors (stimulating protein synthesis and increasing lean body mass) and/or at post-synaptic α receptors involved with conversion of thyroxine to tri-iodothyronine. Xanthines (and aspirin) inhibit negative feedback of released noradrenaline, adenosine and prostaglandins on noradrenaline release from sympathetic nerve terminals[73]. Clinical trials have shown these drugs alone, or in combination, are effective at producing weight loss in obese subjects. In a large 24 week trial, weight loss with a 4.2 MJ/day diet with ephedrine 20 mg and caffeine 200 mg produced more weight loss (0.13–0.14 kg/week) than diet with placebo or ephedrine or caffeine alone[74]. Although in this study there was no increase in heart rate or blood pressure, the expected fall in these measures with weight loss was not seen, suggesting that some of the potential benefit of weight loss may be lost with this form of treatment. In a trial comparing the same ephedrine/caffeine combination with the centrally acting anorectic dexfenfluramine, weight loss was similar after 15 weeks (8.3 ± 5.2 kg vs 6.9 ± 4.3 kg, respectively), but there were significantly more side effects of CNS stimulation in the ephedrine/caffeine treated patients[75]. Long-term treatment for up to 26 months has been reported[76], but only in a few patients and not as part of a randomised controlled trial. Interestingly, much of the effect of phenylpropanolamines on body weight may result from anorexia. One study suggested that 80% of the weight loss in patients treated with the combination could be accounted for by anorexia and decreased food consumption[77].

Atypical beta-adrenoreceptor agonists

The finding of atypical β-adrenoreceptor agonists in 1983[78], soon led to the discovery of atypical receptors (coined β_3 receptors) that mediate the thermogenic effects of sympathomimetic agents, but not the β_1 effects of heart rate stimulation, or β_2 effects on smooth muscle contraction and tremor. The existence of a novel receptor involved in energy expenditure suggested a potentially valuable approach for thermogenic drug development[79]. The field of β_3-adrenoceptor agonists has recently been reviewed by Arch and Wilson[80], and Goldberg and Frishman[81]. In obese rodents, these compounds produce weight loss (from fat) without reducing food intake; in diabetic rodents, they have anti-diabetic effects predominantly through increasing insulin action. Receptors for β_3-adrenoceptor agonists are found predominantly on brown adipocytes, and initially it was thought that the compounds acted to stimulate brown adipose tissue heat production (achieved by the uncoupling of oxidative phosphorylation). However, it seems clear that, in man, skeletal muscle is the main location for thermogenesis induced by these drugs[82], and clinical results have been disappointing. Although two Beecham compounds BRL 26830 and BRL 35135 stimulated metabolic rate and produced weight loss[83,84], the findings were not consistent[85], and the thermogenic effect could not be separated from heat produced by troublesome skeletal muscle tremor[86]. The human β_3 receptor was recently cloned and is known to differ from the rodent receptor. Existing compounds, with activity in rodents, appear to have only poor affinity and specificity for the human receptor. Furthermore, in adult man there is little expression of brown adipose tissue β_3-receptors. At other sites, such as adipose tissue, many of the existing compounds act non-specifically on β_1 and β_2-receptors. More specific compounds are being developed, but are a long way from clinical use.

Drug combinations

Combining drugs with different modes of action is an effective clinical strategy for diseases such as hypertension and diabetes mellitus. It is a strategy that seems logical for obesity treatment, especially since body weight is controlled by factors affecting both energy intake and output. Despite this, only few trials of drug combinations have been reported[87]. The combination of phentermine and fenfluramine has attracted considerable medical and media attention in the US, ever since the report of a 3.5 year trial[88]. All subjects were treated with diet, exercise and behaviour modification, and randomised to a combination of fenfluramine 20 mg + phentermine 15 to 30 mg daily. After a conventional drug versus placebo trial up to 34 weeks, a variety of cross over, drug withdrawal and drug intensification protocols were tested. Interpretation of the 3.5 year results is, therefore, not straightforward, but 26/51 patients completing 190 weeks of treatment maintained a weight loss of 10% initial body weight, with concomitant improvement in serum lipids.

An open trial of this combination involving more than 1000 patients, has been reported by Atkinson[87]. Mean weight loss at 6 months was 16.5 kg and maintained for 18 months. In a separate study, this combination has been used as a maintenance treatment in 96 subjects treated with a very low calorie diet for between 8 and 54 weeks. Mean body weight in 96 subjects fell from 106.6 kg to 89.3 kg on the diet, and to 86.2 kg after 9 months pharmacotherapy (66% patients completing). The combination of phentermine and fenfluramine is well tolerated, although there have been reports that patients suffer from impaired short term memory.

Future possibilities for pharmacological treatment

The rapidly advancing knowledge of the molecular biology of body weight regulation (for example the *ob* gene and its product, leptin) and the neuropharmacological control of ingestive behaviour and energy expenditure holds up the promise of new approaches to obesity treatment.

Rodent models of obesity in which adipose tissue fails to express the *ob* gene (with resulting low levels of leptin) can have their obesity reversed by leptin administration[89]. In obese man, however, leptin levels are high[90], suggesting a receptor defect akin to that seen in the db/db mouse. It, therefore, seems likely that large amounts of leptin would need to be administered to achieve a degree of hyperleptinaemia necessary to 'reset' body weight. However, another approach has been to consider whether giving leptin to offset the fall that is seen with weight loss may be more logical and pragmatic. Human clinical trials are just starting.

Neuropeptide Y (NPY) is the most potent stimulator of food intake, and also increases energy expenditure. Data suggest that leptin, in part, exerts its actions by modulating hypothalamic NPY[91,92]. A number of pharmaceutical companies have developed NPY inhibitors, but it will remain problematic as to how to get such compounds across the blood-brain barrier.

Cholecystokinin (CCK) acts as a physiological satiety factor by reducing meal size[93], whether administered centrally or peripherally. Peripheral CCK-A receptors in the periphery slow gastric emptying and relay to the hypothalamus via the vagus to inhibit feeding. Central CCK-B receptors are found predominantly in the brain. A number of CCK-A promoters are in early development as anti-obesity drugs, and butabindide, which blocks an enzyme that metabolises CCK, is also subject to ongoing research[94]. A number of other peptides that are known to regulate energy metabolism and body weight, and which are thus candidates for pharmacological agonist or antagonist development are reviewed by Levine and Billington[95].

Conclusions

There is a spectrum of body weight from malnourishment with inadequate energy stores, through 'ideal' body weight, to obesity, a state of excessive stores associated with health impairment. Obesity is increasing in our society because human physiology is ill-adapted to changes that have favoured increased energy consumption and decreased energy expenditure. An understanding of the regulation of body weight and energy fluxes is needed if the precise predisposition and causes of excessive fat storage are to be elucidated, and effective treatments developed. At a practical level, it is important for doctors, dietitians and their patients to realise that weight loss can only be achieved by a negative energy balance, and that low levels of energy expenditure do not exist or constitute a bar to achieving this therapeutic goal. The logic of treating obesity with drugs does not differ from treating any other disease or risk factor. Drug treatment should be necessary and more effective than non-drug treatment, and produce a favourable risk benefit ratio. Obesity, as a chronic disease poses particular difficulties for drug treatment. The need for long-term efficacy implies that tolerance or adaptive mechanism must lead to a loss of drug effect. Long-term trials are needed to demonstrate clinical benefit rather than reduction of risk factors or other surrogate measures. There is a growing acceptance of the need and value of drug treatment of obesity, and a growing sophistication of clinical trial design.

References

1   Joint Formulary Committee. *British National Formulary*. London: British Medical Association, Royal Pharmaceutical Society of Great Britain, 1994; 166
2   Bateman DN, Campbell R, Donaldson LJ, Roberts SJ, Smith JM. A prescribing incentive scheme for non-fundholding general practices: an observational study. *BMJ* 1996; **313**: 535–8
3   Rand CSW, Magregor AMC. Morbidly obese patients' perceptions of social discrimination before and after surgery for obesity. *South Med J* 1990; **83**: 1390–5
4   Maddox GL, Liederman V. Overweight as a social disability with medical implications. *J Med Ed* 1969; **44**: 214–20
5   Bray GA. Barriers to the treatment of obesity. *Ann Intern Med* 1991; **115**: 152–3
6   The North American Association for the Study of Obesity. Guidelines for the approval and use of drugs to treat obesity. *Obes Res* 1995; **3**: 473–8
7   Kopelman PG, Finer N, Fox K, Hill AJ, Macdonald IA. ASO Consensus statement on obesity. *Int J Obes* 1994; **18**: 189–91
8   SIGN (Scottish Intercollegiate Guidelines Network). *Obesity in Scotland. Integrating prevention with weight management*. Edinburgh: HMSO, 1996
9   Anonymous Report of the Considerations of the Medicines Commission in October 1995: Proposed prohibition of the sale or supply of medicinal products (anorectic agents) in accordance with section 62 of the Medicines Act 1968. 1996; (Abstract)
10 Kanders BS, Blackburn GL. Health consequences of therapeutic weight loss: reducing primary risk factors. In: Wadden TA, Van Itallie TB (eds) *The Treatment of Morbid Obesity*. New York: Guilford Press, 1992; 213–30
11 Williamson DF, Pamuk ER, Thun M, Flanders D, Byers T, Heath C. Prospective study of intentional weight loss and mortality in never-smoking overweight US white women aged 40-64 years. *Am J Epidemiol* 1995; **141**: 1128–41
12 Han TS, Richmond P, Avenell A, Lean MEJ. Waist circumference reduction and cardiovascular benefits during weight loss in women. *Int J Obes* 1997; **21**: 127–34
13 Goldstein DJ, Potvin JH. Beneficial health effects of modest weight loss. *Int J Obes* 1992; **16**: 397–415
14 Ferner RE. Newly licensed drugs. *BMJ* 1996; **313**: 1157–8
15 Anonymous. Eight basic duties of prescribers. *Drug Ther Bull* 1989; **29**: 65
16 Prentice AM, Jebb SA. Obesity in Britain: obesity or sloth? *BMJ* 1995; **311**: 437–9
17 Blundell JE, Lawton CL. Pharmacological aspects of appetite. In: Stunkard AJ, Wadden TA (eds) *Obesity. Theory and Therapy*. New York: Raven, 1993; 63–76

18 Scoville B. Review of amphetamine-like drugs by the Food and Drug Administration. In: Bray GA (ed) *Obesity in Perspective, Fogarty International Center Series on Preventive Medicine.* Washington DC: US Government Printing Office, 1976; 75–708

19 Campbell DB. Dexfenfluramine: an overview of its mechanisms of action. *Rev Contemp Pharmacother* 1991; 2: 93–113

20 Lessof MH, Myerson A. Benzedrine sulphate as an aid to the treatment of obesity. *N Engl J Med* 1938; 218: 119–24

21 Arch JRS, Piercy V, Thurlby PL. Thermogenic and lipolytic drugs for the treatment of obesity: old ideas and new possibilities. In: Berry EM, Blondheim SH, Eliahou HE, Shafrir E (eds) *Progress in Obesity Research 1990. Proceedings of the 6th International Congress on Obesity.* London: John Libbey, 1987; 300–11

22 Hoekenga MT, O'Dillon RH, Leyland HM. A comprehensive review of dieethylpropion hydrochloride. In: Garattini S, Samanin R (eds) *Central Mechanisms of Anorectic Drugs.* New York: Raven, 1978

23 Carabillo EA. USA drug abuse warning network. In: Garattini S, Samanin R (eds) *Central Mechanisms of Anorectic Drugs.* New York: Raven, 1978

24 Griffiths RR, Brady JV, Bradford LD. Predicting the abuse liability of drugs with animal drug self-administration procedures: psychomotor stimulants and hallucinogens. *Adv Behav Pharmacol* 1979; 2: 163–208

25 Le Riche WH, Csima A. A long-acting appetite suppressant drug studied for 24 weeks in both continuous and sequential administration. *Can Med Assoc J* 1967; 97: 1016–20

26 McKay RH. Long-term use of diethylpropion in obesity. In: Howard AN (ed) *Recent Advances in Obesity Research.* London: Newman, 1975; 388–90

27 Silverstone JT. Intermittent treatment with anorectic drugs. *Practitioner* 1974; 212: 245–52

28 Munro JF, MacCuish AC, Wilson EM, Duncan LJP. Comparison of continuous and intermittent anorectic therapy in obesity. *BMJ* 1968; 1: 352–4

29 Silverstone JT. The place of appetite-suppressant drugs in the treatment of obesity. In: Stunkard AJ, Wadden TA (eds) *Obesity: Theory and Therapy.* New York: Raven, 1993; 275–85

30 McLean Baird I, Howard AN. A double-blind trial of Mazindol using a very low calorie formula diet. *Int J Obes* 1977; 1: 271–8

31 Alger S, Larson K, Boyce VL. Effect of phenylpropanolamine on energy expenditure and weight loss in overweight women. *Am J Clin Nutr* 1993; 57: 120–6

32 Morgan JP, Funderburk FR. Invited commentary: phenylpropanolamine and the medical literature: a thorough reading is required. *Int J Obes* 1990; 14: 569–74

33 Bray GA. Use and abuse of appetite-suppressant drugs in the treatment of obesity (Abstract). *Ann Intern Med* 1993; 119 (Suppl.): 707–13

34 Fuxe K, Hamberger B, Farnebo L, Ogren S. On the *in vivo* and *in vitro* actions of fenfluramine and its derivatives on the central monoamine neurons especially 5-hydroxytryptamine and their relation to the anorectic activity of fenfluramine. *Postgrad Med J* 1975; 51 (Suppl. 5): 35–45

35 Blundell JE, Latham CJ, Moniz E, McArthur RA, Rogers PJ. Structural analysis of the actions of amphetamine and fenfluramine on food intake and feeding behaviour in animals and man. *Curr Med Res Opin* 1979; 6 (Suppl. 1): 34–54

36 Garattini S, Bizzi A, Codegoni AM, Caccia S, Mennini T. Progress report on the anorexia induced by drugs believed to mimic some of the effects of serotonin on the central nervous system. *Am J Clin Nutr* 1992; 55: 160S–5S

37 Pinder RM, Brogden RM, Sawyer PR, Speight TM, Avery GS. Fenfluramine: a review of its pharmacological properties and therapeutic efficacy in obesity and diabetes mellitus. *Drugs* 1975; 10: 241–323

38 Le Douarec JC, Schmitt H, Laubie M. Pharmacological study of dexfenfluramine and its optical isomers. *Arch Int Pharmacodyn* 1966; 161: 206–32

39 McTavish D, Heel RC. Dexfenfluramine: a review of its pharmacological properties and therapeutic potential in obesity. *Drugs* 1992; 43: 713–33

40 Davis R, Faulds D. Dexfenfluramine. An updated review of its therapeutic use in the management of obesity. *Drugs* 1996; 52: 696–724

41 Anonymous. *Obesity Management and Redux.* San Diego: Academic Press, 1997; 1–126

42 Guy-Grand B, Apfelbaum M, Crepaldi G, Gries A, Lefebvre PJ, Turner P. International trial of long-term dexfenfluramine in obesity. *Lancet* 1989; **ii**: 1142–5

43 Guy-Grand B, Apfelbaum M, Crepaldi G, Gries A, Lefebvre PJ, Turner P. Short-term predictors of successful weight loss with dexfenfluramine (dF) (Abstract). *Int J Obes* 1996; **20**: 70

44 Turner P. Dexfenfluramine: its place in weight control. *Drugs* 1990; **39** (Suppl. 3): 53–62

45 Sandage BW, Loar SB, Laudignon N. Review of dexfenfluramine efficacy and tolerability (Abstract). *Int J Obes* 1994; **18** (Suppl. 2): P511

46 Brenot F, Herve P, Petitpretz P, Parent F, Duroux P, Simonneau G. Primary pulmonary hypertension and fenfluramine use. *Br Heart J* 1993; **70**: 537–41

47 Abbenhaim L, Moride Y, Brenot L. Appetite-suppressant drugs and the risk of primary pulmonary hypertension. *N Engl J Med* 1996; **335**: 609–16

48 Manson J, Faich GA. Pharmacotherapy for obesity—do the benefits outweigh the risks? *N Engl J Med* 1996; **335**: 659–60

49 Schutz Y, Munger R, Deriaz O, J quier E. Effect of dexfenfluramine on energy expenditure in man. *Int J Obes* 1992; **16**: S61–S66

50 Breum L, Astrup A, Andersen T *et al*. The effect of long-term dexfenfluramine treatment on 24-hour energy expenditure in man. A double-blind placebo controlled study. *Int J Obes* 1990; **14**: 613–22

51 Munger R, Lavielle R, Arnaud O, Schutz Y, Jéquier E. Enhanced diet-induced thermogenesis in humans after administration of dexfenfluramine. *Proceedings of 2nd European Congress on Obesity* 1988; Abstract

52 Gardiner HM, Freeman CPL, Jessinger DK, Collins SA. Fluvoxamine: an open pilot study in moderately obese female patients suffering from atypical eating disorders and episodes of bingeing. *Int J Obes* 1993; **17**: 301–

53 Samanin R, Garattini S. The neuropharmacology of obesity. *Rev Contemp Pharmacother* 1991; **2**: 53–9

54 Levine LR, Enas GG, Thompson WL *et al*. Use of fluoxetine, a selective serotonin-uptake inhibitor, in the treatment of obesity: a dose-response study (with a commentary by Michael Weintraub). *Int J Obes* 1989; **13**: 635–46

55 Goldstein DJ, Rampey Jr AH, Dornseif BE, Levine LR, Potvin JH. Fluoxetine: a randomised clinical trial in the maintenance of weight loss. *Obes Res* 1993; **1**: 92–8

56 Gray DS, Fujioka K, Devine W, Bray GA. A randomized double-blind clinical trial of fluoxetine in obese diabetics. *Int J Obes* 1992; **16**: S67–S72

57 Darga LL, Carroll-Michals L, Botsford SJ, Lucas CP. Fluoxetine's effect on weight loss in obese subjects. *Am J Clin Nutr* 1991; **54**: 321–5

58 Bray GA, Ryan DH, Gordon D, Heidingsfelder S, Cerise F, Wilson K. A double-blind randomised placebo-controlled trial of sibutramine. *Obes Res* 1996; **4**: 263–70

59 Jones SP, Smith IG, Kelly F, Gray JA. Long-term weight loss with sibutramine. *Int J Obes* 1995; **19** (Suppl. 2): 41

60 Drouin P, Hanotin C, Leutenegger E. Efficacy and tolerability of sibutramine versus dexfenfluramine in obese patients (Abstract). *Int J Obes* 1995; **19** (Suppl. 2): 144

61 Griffiths J, Byrnes AE, Frost G *et al*. Sibutramine in the treatment of overweight non-insulin dependent diabetics (Abstract). *Int J Obes* 1995; **19** (Suppl. 2): 41

62 Hauptman JB, Jeunet FS, Hartmann D. Initial studies in humans with the novel gastrointestinal lipase inhibitor Ro18-0647 (tetrahydrolipstatin). *Am J Clin Nutr* 1992; **55**: 309S–13S

63 Zhi J, Melia AT, Guercolini R *et al*. Retrospective population-based analysis of the dose-response (fecal fat excretion) relationship of orlistat in normal and obese volunteers. *Clin Pharmacol Ther* 1994; **56**: 82–5

64 Drent ML, van der Veen EA. Lipase inhibition: a novel concept in the treatment of obesity. *Int J Obes* 1993; **17**: 241–4

65 Drent ML, Larsson I, William-Olsson T *et al*. Orlistat (Ro18-0647), a lipase inhibitor, in the treatment of obesity: a multiple dose study. *Int J Obes* 1995; **19**: 221–6

66 Finer N, James WPT, Kopelman PG, Lean MEJ, Williams G. Long-term treatment of obesity: a randomised, double-blind, placebo-controlled, multicentre study of orlistat, a gastrointestinal lipase inhibitor. (Submitted for publication)

67 Pavlou KN, Krey S, Steffee WP. Exercise as an adjunct to weight loss and maintenance in moderately obese individuals. *Am J Clin Nutr* 1989; **49**: 1115–23

68 Cawthorne MA. Thermogenic drugs. In: Bjorntorp P, Brodoff BN (eds) *Obesity*. Philadelphia: JB Lippincott, 1992; 762–77

69 Hoogwerf BJ, Nuttall FQ. Long term weight regulation in treated hyperthyroid and hypothyroid patients. *Am J Med* 1984; **30**: 681–6

70 Lessan NG, Finer N. Is hypothyroidism a cause of obesity (Abstract)? *Clin Endocrinol* 1996; **151**: P106

71 Bürgi U, Bürgi-Saville ME, Burgherr J, Clément M, Lauber K. T3 plus high doses of β-blockers: effects on energy intake, body composition, BAT and heart in rats. *Int J Obes* 1990; **14**: 1023–38

72 Malchow-Møller A, Larsen S, Hey H, Stokholm HK, Juhl E, Quaade F. Ephedrine as an anorectic: the story of the 'Elsinore pill'. *Int J Obes* 1981; **5**: 183–8

73 Landsberg L, Young JB. Sympathoadrenal activity and obesity: physiological rationale for the use of adrenergic thermogenic drugs. *Int J Obes* 1993; **17**: S29–S34

74 Astrup A, Breum L, Toubro S, Hein P, Quaade F. The effect and safety of an ephedrine/caffeine compound compared to ephedrine, caffeine and placebo in obese subjects on an energy restricted diet. A double blind trial. *Int J Obes* 1992; **16**: 269–77

75 Breum L, Pederson JK, Ahlstrom F, Frimodt-Moller J. Comparison of an ephedrine/caffeine combination and dexfenfluramine in the treatment of obesity. A double-blind multi-centre trial in general practice. *Int J Obes* 1994; **18**: 99–103

76 Daly P, Krieger DT, Dulloo AG, Young J, Landsberg L. Ephedrine, caffeine and aspirin: safety and efficacy for treatment of human obesity. *Int J Obes* 1993; **17**: S73–S78

77 Astrup A, Buemann B, Christensen NJ *et al*. The effect of ephedrine/caffeine mixture on energy expenditure in obese women. *Metabolism* 1992; **41**: 686–8

78 Arch JRS, Ainsworth AT. Thermogenic and antiobesity activity of a novel β-adrenoreceptor agonist (BRL 26830A) in mice and rats. *Am J Clin Nutr* 1983; **38**: 549–58

79 Arner P. The β3-adreneric receptor — a cause and cure of obesity? *N Engl J Med* 1995; **333**: 382–6

80 Arch JRS, Wilson S. Prospects for β3-adrenoceptor agonists in the treatment of obesity and diabetes. *Int J Obes* 1996; **20**: 191–9

81 Goldberg DE, Frishman WH. *Beta3-Adrenergic Agonism*. New York: Futura, 1995

82 Thurlby PL, Ellis RDM. Differences between the effects of noradrenaline and the β-adrenoreceptor agonist BRL 28410 in brown adipose tissue and hind limb of the anaesthetized rat. *Can J Physiol Pharmacol* 1985; **64**: 1111–4

83 Connacher AA, Jung RT, Mitchell PEG. Weight loss in obese subjects on a restricted diet given BRL 26830A, a new atypical β adrenoceptor agonist. *BMJ* 1988; **296**: 1217–20

84 Connacher AA, Bennet WM, Jung RT, Rennie MJ. Metabolic effects of three weeks administration of the β-adrenoceptor agonist BRL 26830A. *Int J Obes* 1992; **16**: 685–94

85 Chapman BJ, Farquahar DL, Galloway SM, Simpson GK, Munro JF. The effects of a new β-adrenoreceptor agonist BRL 26830A in refractory obesity. *Int J Obes* 1988; **12**: 119–23

86 Connacher AA, Lakie M., Powers N, Elton RA, Walsh EG, Jung RT. Tremor and the anti-obesity drug BRL 26830A. *Br J Clin Pharmacol* 1990; **30**: 613–5

87 Atkinson RL, Blank RC, Loper JF, Schumacher D, Lutes RA. Combined treatment of obesity. *Obes Res* 1995; **3 (Suppl. 4)**: 497S–500S

88 Weintraub M, Sundaresan PR, Madan M *et al*. Long-term weight control: the National Heart, Lung and Blood Institute funded multimodal intervention study (Abstract). *Clin Pharmacol Ther* 1992; **51**: 581–646

89 Rohner-Jeanrenaud F, Jeanrenaud B. Obesity, leptin, and the brain. *N Engl J Med* 1996; **334**: 324–5

90 Considine RV, Sinha MK, Heiman ML, Kriauciunas A, Stephens TW, Nyce MR. Serum immunoreactive-leptin concentrations in normal-weight and obese humans. *N Engl J Med* 1996; **334**: 425–32

91 Stephens TW, Basinski M, Bristow PK, Bue-Valleskey JM, Burgett SG, Craft L. The role of neuropeptide Y in the antiobesity action of the obese gene product. *Nature* 1995; **377**: 530–2

92 Smith FJ, Campfield LA, Moschera JA, Ballon PS, Burn P. Feeding inhibition by neuropeptide Y. *Nature* 1996; **382**: 307

93 Smith GP, Gibbs FP. Satiating effects of cholecystokinin. In: Reeve JRJ, Eysselein V, Solomon TE, Go VLW (eds) *Annals of the New York Academy of Sciences: Cholecystokinin*. New York: New York Academy of Sciences, 1994; 236–41

94 Jack DB. Fighting obesity the Franco-British way. *Lancet* 1996; **347**: 1756

95 Levine AS, Billington CJ. Peptides in the regulation of energy metabolism and body weight. In: Bouchard C, Bray GA (eds) *Regulation of Body Weight: Biological and Behavioural Mechanisms*. Chichester: Wiley, 1996; 179–91

96 Finer N, Craddock D, Lavielle R, Keen H. Dextrofenfluramine in the treatment of refractory obesity. *Curr Ther Res* 1985; **38**: 847–54

97 Enzi G, Crepaldi G, Inelman EM, Bruni R, Baggio B. Efficacy and safety of dexfenfluramine in obese patients: a multicentre study. *Clin Neuropharmacol* 1988; **11** (**Suppl. 1**): S173–S178

98 Finer N, Craddock D, Lavielle R, Keen H. Effect of 6 months therapy with dexfenfluramine in obese patients: studies in the United Kingdom. *Clin Neuropharmacol* 1988; **11** (**Suppl. 1**): 179S–86S

99 Finer N, Finer S, Naoumova RP. Drug therapy after very low calorie diets. *Am J Clin Nutr* 1992; **56**: 195s–98s

100 Noble R. A six-month study of the effects of dexfenfluramine on partially successful dieters. *Curr Ther Res* 1990; **47**: 612–9

101 Mathus-Vliegen EMH, Van de Voore K, Kok AME, Res AMA. Dexfenfluramine in the treatment of sever obesity: a placebo-controlled investigation of the effects on weight loss, cardiovascular risk factors, food intake and eating behaviour. *J Intern Med* 1992; **232**: 119–27

102 Pfohl M, Luft D, Blomberg I, Schmulling R-M. Long-term changes of body weight and cardiovascular risk factors after weight reduction with group therapy and dexfenfluramine. *Int J Obes* 1994; **18**: 391–5

103 Drent ML, Zelissen PMJ, Koppeschaar HPF, Nieuwenhuyzen Kruyzmen AC, Lutterman JA, van der Veen EA. The effect of dexfenfluramine on eating habits in a Dutch ambulatory android overweight population with an overconsumption of snacks. *Int J Obes* 1995; **19**: 299–304

104 O'Connor HT, Richman RM, Steinbeck KS, Caterson ID. Dexfenfluramine treatment of obesity: a double blind trial with post trial follow-up. *Int J Obes* 1995; **19**: 181–9

105 Lucas CP, Sandage BW. Treatment of obese patients with dexfenfluramine: a multicentre, placebo-controlled study. *Am J Ther* 1995; **2**: 962–7

106 Tauber-Lassen E, Damsbo P, Henriksen JE, Palmvig B, Beck-Nielson H. Improvement of glycemic control and weight loss in type 2 (non-insulin-dependent) diabetics after one year of dexfenfluramine treatment (Abstract). *Diabetologia* 1990; **33** (**Suppl.**): A124

107 Stewart GO, Stein GR, Davis TME. Dexfenfluramine in type 2 diabetes: effect on weight and diabetic control. *Med J Aust* 1993; **158**: 167–9

108 Willey KA, Molyneaux LM, Overland JE, Yue DK. The effects of dexfenfluramine on blood glucose control in patients with type 2 diabetes. *Diabetic Med* 1992; **9**: 341–3

109 Manning RM, Jung RT, Leese GP. The comparison of four weight reduction strategies aimed at overweight diabetic patients. *Diabetic Med* 1995; **12**: 409–15

Surgical treatment for morbid obesity

J Kolanowski

Section of Endocrinology and Metabolism, Departments of Physiology and Medicine, Catholic University of Louvain, Brussels, Belgium

Since severe obesity is frequently associated with serious metabolic, cardiovascular and psychological co-morbid conditions, and given the usually unsuccessful results of conservative therapeutic approaches, surgical treatment based on gastric restriction procedures is increasingly recognized as a treatment of choice for morbidly obese persons. Among several surgical approaches designed to promote a substantial loss of weight, two gastric restriction procedures, i.e. the vertical banded gastroplasty and the gastric bypass, have been increasingly used during the past years. Both techniques induce an impressive loss of weight, and are surprisingly well tolerated, even by severely obese persons. The usual 50–75% reduction of initial weight excess, is followed by a clear-cut reduction, or even disappearance of, obesity-related co-morbidity, such as hypertension, diabetes mellitus or sleep apnea syndrome. While serious peri- and postoperative risks are very limited, the intractable vomiting occurring after gastroplasty, and potential sequelae related to iron and calcium malabsorption after the gastric bypass, represent much more frequent complications of the surgical treatment of obesity. There is also a tendency towards a late regain of weight, but the benefit in terms of improvement in the obesity-associated co-morbidity is in general maintained despite this partial increase in weight. Gastric procedures are, therefore, an effective treatment of severe obesity and of its co-morbid conditions. However, careful medical and nutritional supervision is necessary during the follow-up after surgery, to prevent potential nutritional or digestive complications.

Correspondence to:
Prof. J. Kolanowski,
Endocrinology and
Metabolism,
UCL 5530, Av.
Hippocrate 55, B-1200
Brussels, Belgium

There is growing evidence that severe obesity should be considered as a serious morbid condition responsible for increased morbidity and mortality[1–3]. Indeed, life expectancy is reduced proportionally to the severity of the overweight, and obesity-linked morbidity can be considered as the second most preventable cause of death, after cigarette smoking[4]. Obesity-induced health risks result from several co-morbid conditions, such as hypertension, dyslipidaemia, insulin resistance with increased prevalence of non insulin-dependent diabetes mellitus, respiratory dysfunction and some types of cancer[1,2,5]. In addition to these somatic diseases, obesity has a deleterious impact on the quality of life; a less positive mood and anxiety lead frequently to overt depression[6]. It has even been reported that the poor well-being of obese persons is worse than the psychological consequences of several serious morbid states, such as cancer or spinal cord injury[7,8].

It is, therefore, evident that severe obesity should be treated in an effective way, and that obese patients should expect their doctors' help to achieve at least a partial reduction of their overweight. Yet classical conservative treatments, such as dietary and behaviour therapies or the use of anti-obesity drugs, are in general unsuccessful in the long-term. The failure of these treatments is probably partly related to the frequent negative judgement of the obese by physicians[1]. Severely obese persons suffer from prejudice and discrimination; they are frequently considered to be lacking in will-power, lazy, and emotionally unstable, and many physicians share this attitude towards them. It is significant in this respect that nearly 80% of severely obese patients asking for bariatric surgery consider having been previously treated disrespectfully by their doctors because of their weight[7].

This rather dramatic general context of conservative treatment of obesity, as well as an increasing prevalence of obesity over the past decades, prompted the search for a more radical and effective treatment of obesity such as offered by bariatric surgery. While impressive in terms of weight reduction[1,3,5,7], early procedures such as jejuno-ileal bypass induced unacceptable sequelae including chronic diarrhoea with malabsorption, electrolytic disturbances, hepatic failure and deficiencies of fat-soluble vitamins leading ultimately to bone demineralization[5,8,9]. The severity of these complications contributed to the downfall of intestinal bypass surgery, and may explain some of the negative attitudes of physicians towards surgical treatment of the overweight[3,5]. Even today, many physicians are of the opinion that the overall risks and side effects of bariatric surgery do not justify the benefits[9]. However, the interest in developing surgical procedures for the treatment of severe obesity came from the growing recognition of its health consequences, and from the poor long-term results usually seen with medical therapy[1,5,9].

This initially negative opinion concerning the surgical treatment of obesity has been modified by the introduction of gastroplasty and, later on, of gastric bypass. Indeed, gastric partitioning, which considerably limits the amount of ingested food while maintaining the anatomical continuity of the digestive tract, is surprisingly well tolerated, even by extremely obese persons. Moreover, the benefits of gastric surgery are impressive, not only in terms of reduction in weight excess, but also in terms of reduction in co-morbidity and of prevention of further complications of obesity.

The official recognition of gastroplasty, as well as of other forms of gastric bypass, by the National Institutes of Health consensus conference[10,11], as an appropriate treatment for severe obesity associated with serious co-morbid conditions, was followed by an increased use of bariatric surgery, and by further refinement of the originally developed surgical techniques.

Current surgical options

The most popular surgical procedures used for treatment of severe obesity involve gastric partitioning, referred to as gastroplasty, and the gastric bypass (Fig. 1)[13,5]. Both techniques induce a rapid and sustained loss of weight, and are relatively well tolerated[1,5,12]. Only some general features of these techniques will be described here, while emphasis will be laid essentially on the beneficial effects and potential sequelae.

Gastroplasties

These procedures create a small gastric pouch, which is drained through a narrow calibrated stoma[5,13]. The intake of solids is, therefore, considerably limited. Patients appear not to experience hunger, and rapidly feel full, even after a small meal. These procedures do not involve gastric resection and maintain the anatomical and functional continuity

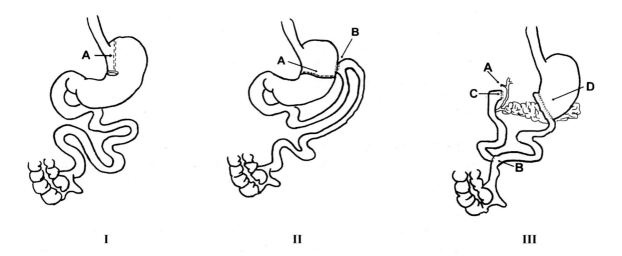

| I | II | III |

Fig. 1 (I) Vertical banded gastroplasty. A staple line (A) to produce a 20 to 30 ml pouch is applied to the stomach and a Gortex band produces an outlet diameter of about 1 cm. (II) Gastric bypass. A loop of small bowel is brought up to drain an isolated section of stomach (B) produced by stapling (A). (III) Scopinaro bilio-pancreatic diversion. The stomach is divided and resected and anastamosed to a Y loop of intestine (D). The gall bladder is removed (A), and the duodenum closed (C); the jejunum is anastamosed to the ileum (B).

of the gastro-intestinal tract. Digestion and intestinal absorption are, therefore, normally maintained, and the loss of weight is due solely to a very restricted energy intake[3,5].

Vertical banded gastroplasty   Vertical banded gastroplasty, introduced by Mason in 1982[14], rapidly became the most popular technique of gastric restriction, and is still widely used. This technique involves the stapled partition of the stomach creating a small upper pouch of 30 ml, which empties to the remaining part of the stomach through a narrow outlet with diameter calibrated from 8 to 10 mm, and reinforced by a Gortex band, or by a similar prosthetic material[3,5,13]. Because of the limited capacity of the gastric pouch, the amount of ingested food before rapid onset of satiety is considerably limited[3]. This induces, obviously, a rapid loss of weight, which occurs mainly during the first 6 months after the operation[5,8,15]. The peri-and early postoperative mortality is lower than 1%, while the immediate postoperative complications are in general limited to wound infection encountered, however, only in 2% of patients according to the recent report of Mason and Doherty[8]. In other series, wound problems have been seen in 23% of patients[9]. Intractable vomiting represents a more frequent postoperative complication, caused by too rapid intake of solids, rather than by stenosis of the stoma[3,5]. Frequent vomiting associated with gastro-oesophageal reflux may, however, occur in some patients, as a result of stomal stenosis; this may prove refractory even to multiple attempts at endoscopic balloon catheter dilation[16]. Late failure in terms of insufficient loss of weight, or even of weight regain, may result either from an excessive ingestion of high-calorie liquids and sweet foods, or from staple disruption. The later is usually followed by a suddenly increased capacity of solid food ingestion, and may be easily evidenced by radiography.

Horizontal gastroplasty   Horizontal gastroplasty may involve a stapled horizontal partition of the stomach, but is more frequently realized by encircling the upper stomach with a plastic collar[3,5]. Some surgeons are using an inflatable prosthetic device, allowing a variable calibration of the outlet to the lower part of the stomach[3]. This procedure may be relatively easily performed by laparoscopy, but it is, in general, considered as mechanically unreliable and gives rather disappointing results[3,5]. Insufficient loss of weight is frequently related to the distension of the thin-walled gastric fundus[8]. In addition, reflux oesophagitis is relatively common after this kind of surgery. Since gastric restriction surgery performed by laparoscopy is followed by a shorter and less cumbersome postoperative recovery, some surgeons are using this technique to perform not only gastric banding but also vertical banded gastroplasty[17]. These are, however, technically difficult operations, and the limited experience in this field does not allow a conclusion as to whether this approach represents a real advantage with respect to open surgery.

If vertical banded gastroplasty is followed by complications, such as intractable vomiting with gastro-oesophageal reflux, staple line disruption or inadequate loss of weight, some authors advocate conversion of complicated or failed gastroplasty to gastric bypass[16]. This opinion is not shared by Mason[18] who considers that, in the case of staple disruption, the simplest revision is to restaple the pouch, and that vertical banded gastroplasty not followed by a stenosis of the outlet, is amongst the best of antireflux operations.

Gastric bypass

This surgical procedure creates a larger pouch, emptied by an anastomosis directly into the jejunum, thus bypassing the duodenum. It is considered now as the most effective and safe surgery for morbid obesity[3,5,9]. This technique induces weight loss by combining restricted intake and a moderate degree of malabsorption[1,3,5]. There is no doubt that the initial loss of weight is greater after this procedure than following gastroplasty[3,8,9,19]. The gastric pouch is separated from the excluded part of the stomach by stapling, and drained through a relatively large stoma directly into a jejunal loop in a Roux-en-Y arrangement[8]. Thus, one limb of a Y-shaped reconstruction of jejunum allows the drainage of the gastric pouch, while the bile and pancreatic juice are evacuated by the second limb of the Y structure. Since hypertonic contents of the stomach rapidly enter the small bowel, patients frequently experience a dumping syndrome consisting of weakness and sweating after a carbohydrate-rich meal[1,3,5,8]. This may obviously discourage them to consume sweet foods; hence the opinion[3] that this type of gastrojejunal surgery is particularly indicated for obese patients considered as 'sweet eaters'. It should be stressed, however, that by bypassing the duodenum, this kind of surgery may cause malabsorption of iron and calcium, increasing the risk of anaemia, osteoporosis and hip fracture[8,9].

Biliopancreatic diversion A particular form of gastric bypass, referred to as biliopancreatic diversion, introduced in 1968 by Scopinaro[20], was designed to bypass a large part of the intestine with a concomitant resection of the excluded part of the stomach to decrease the risk of gastric ulcer. While the volume of the remaining gastric pouch is much larger than in other procedures, and may vary from 200–500 ml, the loss of weight is essentially due to intestinal malabsorption. This procedure seems very effective in terms of loss of weight, but frequently induces protein malnutrition and other metabolic complications[8,20]. It is, therefore, not surprising that the extent of weight loss after this kind of surgery is proportional to the length of the intestinal bypass and, thus, to the severity of malabsorption and risks of late complications[5,8].

Long-term benefits of gastric surgery

The loss of weight induced by gastric restriction procedures is due solely to decreased energy intake. Given the considerably reduced capacity of gastric pouch, the ingestion of energy is limited usually during the first three postoperative months to 400–600 kcal/day[15]. Dietary records indicate that, during this initial period after gastroplasty, protein and fat intake is less than 30 g/day, the remaining energy consisting of carbohydrates ingested mainly as sweet liquids and semi-solid foods. Protein intake is limited by the aversion towards meats, which may persist for several months. The intake of protein is provided by dairy products and eggs and, later on, by poultry and fish. Patients are instructed to take frequent and small meals and, to prevent vomiting, to eat slowly and to avoid drinking during meals[3].

As a result of these radical changes in eating habits, a rapid loss of weight usually averaging 20–25 kg develops during the first 3 months after operation[8,15]. At least 70% of the weight lost during this period is accounted for by a reduction of fat mass, the remaining loss corresponding to fat-free mass (lean tissue, intracellular and extra-cellular water). While the loss of lean tissue, resulting from a negative nitrogen balance, which averages 2–4 g of nitrogen per day, occurs mainly during the first weeks after surgery, the water lost during this period is usually recovered after 2–3 months[21]. Later on, weight loss corresponds solely to the reduction of body fat, thus to the essential goal of the treatment. Loss of weight continues, albeit at a slower rate, during the following 3 months, and corresponds, at 6 months after surgery, to 40–50% of the pre-operative weight excess[15]. At this time, the adaptation of eating habits and improved gastric tolerance allows a progressive increase and variety in consumption of solid foods, with a concomitant increase in protein, fat as well as mineral and vitamin intake. Energy intake thereafter progressively increases, and at 1 year after surgery averages 800–1000 kcal/day[15]. This obviously reduces the loss of weight, which frequently ceases 12–18 months after gastroplasty, by when the loss of weight may account for to 60%, or even to 75%, of the initial excess of weight[8,15].

The loss of weight during the first year after surgery is proportional to the degree of the pre-operative obesity, and depends largely on the frequency of the follow-up visits[3]. It may be considerably slower in obese subjects who consume large amounts of sweets and high-energy liquid foods rich in sugars and fat. According to some authors[5,16], vertical banded gastroplasty is not a suitable intervention in these subjects, and gastric bypass offers them much better postoperative results. Indeed, the gastric bypass procedure is followed by rapid emptying of the gastric pouch into the small bowel with ensuing aversion to sweets, due to the dumping syndrome[3,9,16].

Long-term loss of weight 2 years after surgery is variable and depends largely on eating habits. Despite some tendency toward a weight regain, some reports indicate that at least a 50% reduction of the pre-operative weight excess may be maintained for periods as long as 10–15 years after surgery[8,9,12]. Weight loss is greater and maintained for longer periods after gastric bypass or biliopancreatic diversion than after gastroplasty[9]. This is not surprising since the former procedures induce a variable degree of intestinal malabsorption, as will be discussed later on.

According to recent results published by Mason and Doherty[8], at 5 years after vertical banded gastroplasty, 48% of patients achieve a reduction of 51% or more of the initial weight excess. Modest success, defined as a loss of excess weight ranging between 25% and 50%, is obtained in 30% of patients. 22% can be considered to fail, due either to the insufficient loss of weight (16%) or to complications requiring revisional surgery (6%).

The impressive loss of weight, which usually follows gastric restriction procedure, is associated in most patients with a considerable improvement in the quality of life[1,5,9]. The most important benefit, however, relates to a rapid improvement in several co-morbid conditions, such as hypertension, hyperlipidaemia, hyperuricaemia and glucose intolerance[3,5,15,22,23]. The latter results from a significant increase in the sensitivity to insulin[15,24], with the clearcut improvement in glucose tolerance normalising hyperglycaemia in most previous non insulin-dependent diabetic subjects. Respiratory function is also improved, with significant regression or even disappearance of the sleep apnea syndrome[3]. There is also a rapid amelioration of abnormal cardiac function[25]. According to Stunkard[26], the most striking indication of improvement in health is the increased life expectancy, but results from long-term follow-up studies are needed to confirm this. The Swedish Obese Subjects (SOS) study was designed to address this important question[6]. The preliminary data arising from this study are impressive: a considerable reduction in the incidence of diabetes mellitus and in cardiovascular complications.

While weight is seldom normalised, the partial reduction of the overweight is, in general, sufficient to correct many co-morbid conditions[3,15]. These improvements are frequently associated with increased work capacity, hence a better rehabilitation into professional and social life.

Gastric surgery — related risks and complications

As already mentioned, the peri-operative mortality and early complications are extremely low, and the expected improvement in health considerably reduces the risk-to-benefit ratio. However, late gastric and nutritional complications may be relatively serious in some patients, largely depending on the type of operation as well as on the frequency and quality of the medical, psychological and nutritional follow-up.

Although vertical banded gastroplasty is well tolerated by most patients, some reports indicated a relatively high frequency of intractable vomiting related to gastro-oesophageal reflux [27]. This complication rarely results from stenosis of the gastric pouch outlet, and is usually secondary to too rapid eating[3]. Another, relatively frequent, complication is disruption of the staple line[3,8,9]. This complication, usually followed by a sudden increase in eating capacity, with ensuing regain of weight, may need revisional surgery: either restapling of the gastric pouch, or the conversion of gastroplasty into gastric bypass. An intragastric migration of the polypropylene band restricting the gastric outlet, or ulceration of the stoma, have also been reported, but remain rare. Nutritional deficiencies are seldom encountered after vertical banded gastroplasty, despite the considerable restriction of nutrient intake, described by some authors[28] as a state of 'starvation in the midst of plenty'.

The most frequent nutritional deficiency is insufficient intake of iron and proteins, and thus anaemia[29]. While low serum iron and ferritin levels are frequently observed after gastroplasty[15], there is usually no fall in hemoglobin level or in the number of blood red cells. Thiamine deficiency, with neurological sequelae, may also occur[28,29], especially in subjects suffering from intractable vomiting. If intravenous glucose is administered, it may exacerbate the problem by increasing demand for thiamine[28]. The most threatening early complication of gastric bypass is an anastomotic leak, which, according to some reports[9], occurs in up to 4% of patients. More frequent complications include anaemia, vitamin and mineral deficiencies and dehydration[9,29].

Nutritional deficiencies are much more frequent after gastric bypass than after gastroplasty[8,9], since the duodenum, the site of iron and calcium absorption, is bypassed. As well as iron and calcium depletion, low serum vitamin B12 and vitamin B1 concentrations are more frequently seen after gastric bypass than following simple gastric partitioning procedures[16,29,30]. These nutritional deficiencies are even more frequent and serious after the biliopancreatic diversion, which bypasses not only the duodenum but also a large proportion of the small bowel[20]. The excluded limbs are much longer following this type of surgery and, in addition, a large part of the stomach is removed (to decrease the risk of gastric ulcer)[20]. Obviously this procedure considerably increases the risk of protein, mineral and vitamin deficiencies, a risk further aggravated by a tendency for patients to develop chronic diarrhoea[9,20]. To prevent the serious risk of malnutrition, especially anaemia and bone demineralization, patients should be supplemented early after the surgery with iron, calcium as well as with vitamins B1 and B12. According to the recent report by Scopinaro[20], the impressive loss of weight, averaging a 78% reduction of weight excess at 2 years and still 70% reduction 15 years after surgery, may be associated with severe nutritional deficiencies. Indeed, protein malnutrition is observed in 12% of patients, most by developing at the same time as iron, calcium and vitamin deficiencies which occur in 35% of patients[20].

Nutritional supplementation after gastric bypass procedures, and especially after biliopancreatic diversion, is therefore mandatory. The risk of peripheral neuropathy and Wernicke's encephalopathy[28,29], necessitates supplementation with vitamin B1. To avoid calcium depletion and osteoporosis, Scopinaro advises a daily supplement of 2 g calcium (often not taken by patients), as well as a monthly intramuscular injection of 400,000 IU vitamin D[20]. Despite these preventive measures, 7% of patients undergoing this surgical treatment develop bone demineralization, usually between the second and fifth postoperative years[19]. Since vitamin B12, in its protein-bound form, is poorly absorbed in these patients, Rhode[30] has recently suggested daily administration of the crystalline form of vitamin B12 at very high dosage. Indeed, at least 350 µg of crystalline vitamin B12 are necessary to normalize the serum levels of this vitamin, and a dosage as high as 500 µg/day has been recommended[16]. Monthly vitamin B12 injections may be substituted for oral administration. Gastric outlet obstruction and severe nutritional deficiency may necessitate revisional surgery, consisting usually of conversion into the vertical banded gastroplasty[12].

In addition to nutritional deficiencies, the restrictive eating behaviour and marked loss of weight which occurs after gastric surgery may lead exceptionally to anorexia nervosa[31]. This complication may occur despite a careful psychiatric assessment prior to bariatric surgery[31]. It is, in general, considered that the pre-operative evaluation of psychiatric status is of little value in predicting the magnitude of weight loss after gastroplasty[1,31,32]. Albeit the gastric procedures are successful in producing weight loss, gastroplasty does not change abnormalities of eating behaviour that existed before surgery[3,32]. Indeed, recent evaluation of a large number of patients who had undergone gastroplasty[32], indicated that surgery did not attenuate disturbances of eating behaviour, such as bulimia nervosa or 'night eating syndrome'. This is of importance, since individuals who crave sweets and consume large quantities of soft foods and sweet liquids, may not lose weight satisfactorily after either gastroplasty or gastric bypass procedures. The available data indicate that co-morbid psychiatric disorders are not improved by weight-reduction surgery, despite the usual substantial improvement in psychosocial functioning[5,32]. This clearly indicates that patients undergoing bariatric surgery should be followed closely from a psychological, or even psychiatric, standpoint for several years after operation. It appears, nevertheless, that the psychiatric status and personality disturbance do not seem to affect the weight loss outcome of bariatric surgery[8,32]. Furthermore, psychologists or psychiatrists cannot predict reliably whether dietary compliance will be satisfactory or not after surgery, nor whether the patient will improve or deteriorate from a psychological point of view.

General conclusions and indications for gastric surgery

There is an increasing body of evidence suggesting that gastric restriction procedures, such as vertical banded gastroplasty and the gastric bypass, represent an appropriate, and sometimes the only effective therapy for morbidly obese subjects. While the surgeon should inform the morbidly obese patient that surgery is unlikely to normalise body weight, the patient can be advised that even a moderate loss of weight will be sufficient to greatly reduce the obesity associated co-morbidity. When properly conducted conservative approaches fail to produce significant weight reduction in the overweight, the treatment of choice is surgery. Less severely obese patients may also be considered for surgical treatment, if they suffer from significant co-morbidity.

The choice of procedure is important. According to current opinion, patients who consume large amounts of sugars or carbohydrates are more suited to gastric bypass, because symptoms of dumping may be important in contributing to a drastic reduction of energy intake. In contrast, in so called 'big eaters', the vertical banded gastroplasty, which induces early satiety even after a small meal, seems to be a preferred surgical option.

The impressive loss of weight which follows gastric restriction surgery is in general well tolerated and followed by a considerable improvement or even disappearance of many co-morbid conditions, such as hypertension, respiratory and cardiac dysfunction, abnormal serum lipid profile and non insulin-dependent diabetes mellitus. Gastric restriction surgery may be, therefore, proposed as a treatment for obesity if the following criteria are fulfilled:

1. The patient should be morbidly obese with a body mass index (BMI) above 40 kg/m^2
2. The patient with a BMI between 36 and 40 kg/m^2 may also be considered for gastric surgery if there are serious obesity-associated co-morbidities
3. Obesity should have been present for at least 5 years, and be refractory to several attempts at reducing weight by non-surgical methods
4. There should be no history of alcoholism or major psychiatric disorders. In this respect, it appears that the current mental state of the patient is more relevant than a past history of depression or minor psychiatric disorders.

Providing patients are appropriately selected both on the above criteria and also on the nature of the co-existing abnormalities of eating behaviour, gastric restriction surgery represents a significant progress in the treatment of severe obesity and of its health-threatening complications.

References

1   Stunkard AJ. Current views on obesity. *Am J Med* 1996; **100**: 230–6
2   Sjöström L. Morbidity of severely obese subjects. *Am J Clin Nutr* 1992; **55** (**Suppl.**): 508S–15S
3   Sagar PM. Surgical treatment of morbid obesity. *Br J Surg* 1995; **82**: 732–9
4   McGinnis JM, Foege WH. Actual causes of death in the United States. *JAMA* 1993; **270**: 2207–12
5   Kral JG. Overview of surgical techniques for treating obesity. *Am J Clin Nutr* 1992; **55** (**Suppl.**): 552S–5S
6   Sullivan M, Karlsson J, Sjöström L *et al.* Swedish obese subjects (SOS) — an intervention study of obesity. Baseline evaluation of health and psychosocial functioning in the first 1743 subjects examined. *Int J Obes* 1993; **17**: 503–12
7   Rand CSW, Macgregor AMC. Successful weight loss following obesity surgery and perceived liability of morbid obesity. *Int J Obes* 1991; **15**: 577–9
8   Mason EE, Doherty C. Surgery. In: Stunkard AJ, Wadden TA (eds) *Obesity, Theory and Therapy*, 2nd edn. New York: Raven, 1993; 313–25
9   Shikora SA, Benotti PN, Forse RA. Surgical treatment of obesity. In: Blackburn GL, Kanders BS (eds) *Obesity, Pathophysiology, Psychology and Treatment*. New York: Chapman & Hall, 1994; 264–82
10 NIH Consensus Development Conference Panel. Gastrointestinal surgery for severe obesity. *Ann Intern Med* 1991; **115**: 956–61

11 Editorial: Gastrointestinal surgery for severe obesity: NIH Cons. Dev. Conf. Statement. *Am J Clin Nutr* 1992; **55** (**Suppl.**): 615S–9S

12 Reinhold RB. Late results of gastric bypass surgery for morbid obesity. *J Am Coll Nutr* 1994; **13**: 326–31

13 Ashley S, Bird DL, Sugden G, Royston CM. Vertical banded gastroplasty for the treatment of morbid obesity. *Br J Surg* 1993; **80**: 1421–3

14 Mason EE. Vertical banded gastroplasty for obesity. *Arch Surg* 1982; **117**: 701–6

15 Kolanowski J. Gastroplasty for morbid obesity: the internist's view. *Int J Obes* 1995; **19** (**Suppl. 3**): S61–S65

16 Sugerman HJ, Kellum JM, De Maria EJ, Reines HD. Conversion of failed or complicated vertical banded gastroplasty to gastric bypass in morbid obesity. *Am J Surg* 1996; **171**: 263–7

17 Lönroth H, Dalenbäck J, Haglind E *et al*. Vertical banded gastroplasty by laparoscopic technique in the treatment of morbid obesity. *Surg Laparoscopy Endoscopy* 1996; **6**: 102–7

18 Mason EE. Editorial comments. *Am J Surg* 1996; **171**: 267–9

19 Salmon PA, McArdle MO. The rationale and results of gastroplasty/distal gastric bypass. *Obes Surg* 1992; **2**: 61–8

20 Scopinaro N, Gianetta E, Adami GF *et al*. Biliopancreatic diversion for obesity at eighteen years. *Surgery* 1996; **119**: 261–8

21 Kolanowski J, Martinelli M. Changes in body composition and in energy expenditure after gastroplasty in morbidly obese patients. *Int J Obes* 1996; **20** (**Suppl. 4**): 134

22 Gleysteen JJ. Results of surgery: long term effects on hyperlipidemia. *Am J Clin Nutr* 1992; **55** (**Suppl.**): 591S–3S

23 Von Schenck H, Wallentin L, Lennmarken C, Larsson J. Lipoprotein metabolism following gastroplasty in obese women. *Scand J Clin Lab Invest* 1992; **52**: 269–74

24 Burstein R, Epstein Y, Charuzi I *et al*. Glucose utilization in morbidly obese subjects before and after weight loss by gastric bypass operation. *Int J Obes* 1995; **19**: 558–61

25 Alpert MA, Terry BE, Lambert CR *et al*. Factors influencing left ventricular systolic function in non hypertensive morbidly obese patients, and effect of weight loss induced by gastroplasty. *Am J Cardiol* 1993; **71**: 733–7

26 Stunkard AJ, Stinnett JL, Smoller JW. Psychological and social aspects of the surgical treatment of obesity. *Am J Psychiatry* 1986; **143**: 412–29

27 Kim CH, Sarr MG. Severe reflux esophagitis after vertical banded gastroplasty for treatment of morbid obesity. *Mayo Clin Proc* 1992; **67**: 33–5

28 Seehra H, MacDermott N, Lascelles RG, Taylor TV. Wernicke's encephalopathy after vertical banded gastroplasty for morbid obesity. *BMJ* 1996; **312**: 434

29 Albina JE, Stone WM, Bates M, Felder ME. Catastrophic weight loss after vertical banded gastroplasty: malnutrition and neurological alterations. *J Parent Enteral Nutr* 1988; **12**: 619–20

30 Rhode BM, Arseneau P, Cooper BA *et al*. Vitamin B-12 deficiency after gastric surgery for obesity. *Am J Clin Nutr* 1996; **63**: 103–9

31 Boone OB, Bashi R, Berry EM. Anorexia nervosa following gastroplasty in the male: two cases. *Int J Eating Disorders* 1996; **19**: 105–8

32 Hsu LKG, Betancourt S, Sullivan SP. Eating disturbances before and after vertical banded gastroplasty: a pilot study. *Int J Eating Disorders* 1996; **19**: 23–34

Index

Apoptosis

Scientific Editor

Andrew H Wyllie